M. Ackenheil · B. Bondy · R. Engel · M. Ermann · N. Nedopil (Eds.)
Implications of Psychopharmacology to Psychiatry

Springer
Berlin
Heidelberg
New York
Barcelona
Budapest
Hong Kong
London
Milan
Paris
Tokyo

M. Ackenheil · B. Bondy · R. Engel · M. Ermann
N. Nedopil (Eds.)

Implications of Psychopharmacology to Psychiatry

Biological, Nosological, and Therapeutical Concepts

With 35 Figures and 34 Tables

Springer

Prof. Dr. M. Ackenheil
Priv.-Doz. Dr. B. Bondy
Prof. Dr. R. Engel
Prof. Dr. M. Ermann
Prof. Dr. N. Nedopil
Ludwig-Maximilians-Universität München
Psychiatrische Klinik und Poliklinik
Nußbaumstraße 7
80336 München

ISBN-13:978-3-642-64683-6 e-ISBN-13:978-3-642-61076-9
DOI: 10.1007/978-3-642-61076-9

Die Deutsche Bibliothek – CIP-Einheitsaufnahme
Implications of psychopharmalcology to psychiatry : biological, nosological, and therpeutical concepts ; with 34 tables / M. Ackenheil ... (ed.). – Berlin ; Heidelberg ; New York ; Barcelona ; Budapest ; Hong Kong ; London ; Milan ; Paris ; Tokyo : Springer, 1996
ISBN-13:978-3-642-64683-6
NE: Ackenheil, Manfred [Hrsg.]

Softcover reprint of the hardcover 1st edition 1996

Product Liability: The publisher can give no guarantee for information about drug dosage and application thereof contained in this book. In every individual case the respective user must check ist accuracy by consulting other pharmaceutical literature.
The use of registered names, trademarkes, etc. in this publication does not imply, even in the absence of a specific statement, that such names are exempt from the relevant protective laws and regulations and therefore free for general use.

Typesetting: FotoSatz Pfeifer GmbH, 82166 Gräfelfing
SPIN: 10514069 25/3130 – 5 4 3 2 1 0 – Printed on acid-free paper

Preface

The discovery of chlorpromazine for the specific treatment of schizophrenic symptoms and, later on, of imipramine for the specific treatment of depressive symptoms marked a new milestone in clinical psychiatry and basic neuroscience 40 years ago. The exploration of biochemical mechanisms of action of these psychotropic drugs created new theories on the pathophysiology of psychiatric disorders, such as the dopamine hypothesis of schizophrenia and the catecholamine and serotonin hypotheses of depression. Thus the discovery of these biological treatments had a major impact on natural science-oriented research. Biological psychiatry as we know it today has its origin in these psychopharmacological drugs and influences many disciplines in psychiatry.

It was a fortunate coincidence that Hans Hippius, whose 70th birthday we celebrated this year with an international symposium, started his professional career during this time in the 1950s. He was one of the early pioneers in clinical psychopharmacological research and enthusiastic about both the scientific and the therapeutic prospects of the new psychotropic drugs. He has worked in this field for more than three decades and has made many lasting contributions to biological psychiatry. Among the many activities, his contributions in the development of the new atypical antipsychotic drug clozapine should be mentioned.

Hanns Hippius has been active in many international societies and the occasion of his birthday brought together leading experts in the field of psychopharmacology, biological psychiatry, and related disciplines. They presented and discussed their views and theories on psychiatric disorders. This Festschrift presents future perspectives in drug development, genetic research in psychiatry, nosological and diagnostic concepts, as well as strategies for a more specific treatment of the different psychiatric disorders. The implications of psychopharmacology to psychiatry are elaborated. The authors, internationally prominent experts, give broad insight into their research and into the clinical perspectives of psychiatry. Many of them are prominent members of the European College of Neuropsychopharmacology, of which Hanns Hippius is a honorary member.

We thank the authors of this Festschrift very much for their contributions.

M. Ackenheil, B. Bondy
München, September 1995

List of Authors

Professor Dr. Jules Angst, Psychiatric University Hospital Zürich, Research Department, P.O. Box 68, Lenggstraße 31, CH-8029 Zürich, Switzerland

Professor Arvid Carlsson, Depatment of Pharmacology, University of Göteborg, Medicinaregatan 7, S-41390 Göteborg, Sweden

Dr. Elliot S. Gershon, Chief, Clinical Neurogenetics Branch, National Institute of Mental Health, 10-3N218, Bethesda, Maryland 20892, U.S.A.

Dr. Frederik K. Goodwin, The George Washington Unviversity, Medical Center, Department of Psychiatry, 2300 I Street, NW Rm 514, Washington D.C. 20337, U.S.A.

Prof. Dr. Dr. Heinz Häfner, Zentralinstitut für Seelische Gesundheit, Postfach 12 21 20, 68072 Mannheim

Professor John M. Kane, Hillside Hospital, Department of Psychiatry, 75-79 263rd Street, Glen Oaks, N.Y. 11004, U.S.A.

Professor Otto F. Kernberg, The New York Hospital, Cornell Medical Center, 21 Bloomingdale Road, White Planes, N.Y. 10605, U.S.A.

Dr. Donald F. Klein, Director of Research, New York State Psychiatric Institute, 722 West 168th Street, New York, N.Y. 10032, U.S.A.

Professor Malcolm Lader, Institute of Psychiatry, De Crespigny Park, Denmark Hill, London SE5 8AF, U.K.

Professor Julien Mendlewicz, Free University of Brussels, Erasme Hospital, Department of Psychiatry, Route de Lennick 808, B-1070 Belgium

Professor H.-J. Möller, Psychiatric Hospital, University of Munich, Nussbaumstr. 7, D-80336 Munich

Professor Stuart Montgomery, St. Mary's Hospital Medical School, Academic Department of Psychiatry, Praed Street, London W2 1NY, U.K.

Dr. Steven Paul, Vice President, Lilly Research Laboratories, Indianapolis, Indiana 46285, U.S.A.

Professor Herman van Praag, Academic Hospital Maastricht, Department of Psychiatry, P. Delylaan 25, 6202 AZ Maastricht, The Netherlands

Professor Giorgio Racagni, Center of Neuropharmacology, University of Milan, Via Balzaretti 9, I-20133 Milan, Italy

Prof. Dr. M. L. Rao, Psychiatrische Klinik und Poliklinik der Universität Bonn, Sigmund-Freud-Str. 25, 53105 Bonn

Sir Martin Roth, Professor Emeritus of Psychiatry, Trinity College, Cambridge CB2 2 TQ, U.K.

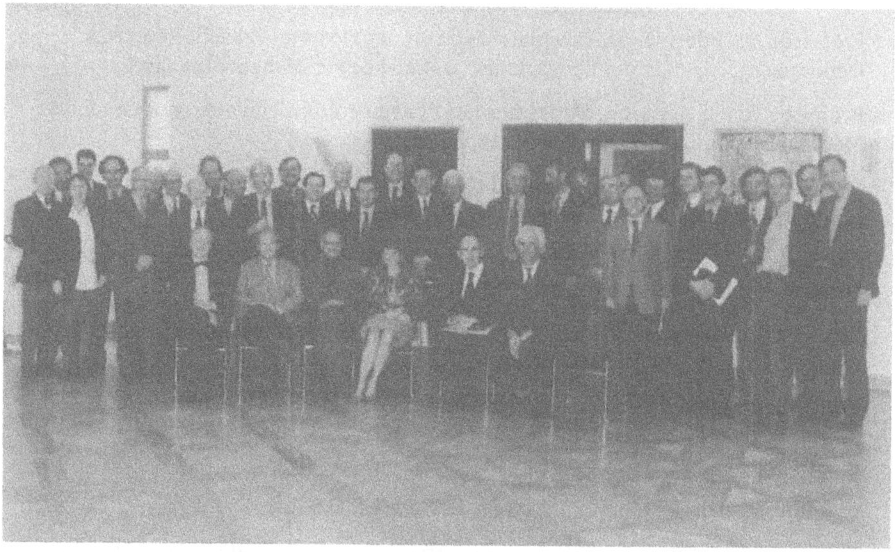

Sitting, from left to right: A. Carlsson, J. Mendlewicz, J. Angst, B. Bondy, Sir M. Roth, M. Ackenheil

Standing, from left to right, first row: G. Kurtz, P. Buchheim, O. Kernberg, H. van Praag, J. Racagni, S. Montgomery, N. Sartorius, D. Klein, H. Häfner, M. Lader, W. Greil, W. Guenther, P. Simon, H. Dilling

Standing, second row: J. Martinius, R. Cohen, A. Erfurth, R. Steinberg, P. Berner, E. Rüther, H. Helmchen, G. Laakmann, E. Gershon, H. Hippius, R. Engel, U. Hegerl, H. Sass, D. van Zerssen

Contents

Neurotransmitter Interactions Important for Schizophrenia

A. Carlsson

Introduction

Hanns Hippius and I belong to the same generation of medical students, and thus we were able to witness the revolution of psychiatry that was initiated by the discovery of neuroleptics. Already as a schoolboy and later as a medical student I had the opportunity of observing the bizarre appearance and behavior of patients in a mental hospital in the 1930s and 1940s. And of course Hanns Hippius made similar observations. Inevitably both of us, as everybody else at that time, were astounded by the change that these patients underwent after the introduction of chlorpromazine, following the report by Delay and Deniker in 1952 [1]. The therapeutic response to neuroleptic treatment during the early days after its introduction was perhaps more dramatic and spectacular than can be seen today, because at that time most schizophrenic patients in a mental hospital were presumably good responders, whereas today the percentage of responders among hospitalized patients may be lower, since the good responders are less likely to be hospitalized at any given time.

I have had the privilege of meeting and interacing with Hanns Hippius and have benefited from his wisdom and thorough knowledge numerous times over more than three decades. At this time I wish to focus on only one occasion – the International Symposium on Antipsychotic Drugs held in Stockholm in September, 1974. Hanns was given the task of summarizing the state of the art at that time, viewed from the perspective of a clinical psychiatrist [2]. I was impressed by his review, and after rereading it now, two decades later, I am still impressed. Hanns focused on the then controversial issue of the relation between antipsychotic and extrapyramidal drug effects and demonstrated convincingly that there is no close linkage between the two. The most compelling argument came from the experience regarding clozapine gleaned for more than 8 years by himself and a number of other European psychiatrists. It is indeed remarkable how well the properties of clozapine were already characterized at that time. Obviously Hanns had contributed very much to the accumulation of this important information and its far-reaching implications. Thanks to the work of numerous other psychiatrists this contribution was later corroborated and extended. Needless to say, this is just one example of the profound impact of Hanns Hippius's work extending over several decades.

The Dopamine Hypothesis of Schizophrenia – and Beyond

The present chapter will focus on the possible role of neurotransmitter aberrations in our understanding of schizophrenia and its therapeutic implications.

Although the dopamine hypothesis of schizophrenia has served us well for several decades, there is now a general trend to try to widen the perspective and look into alternative pathogenetic mechanisms. For one thing it seems likely that schizophrenia is a heterogeneous group of disorders based on different etiologic and pathogenetic mechanisms. Moreover, the dopamine hypothesis rests almost entirely on indirect, pharmacologic evidence, and not even this evidence is unambiguous. For example, antidopaminergic agents are not always efficacious in schizophrenia, and the symptomatology of schizophrenia is mimicked not only by dopaminergic agonists but also, for example, by phencylidine (PCP) [3], an antiglutamatergic agent blocking the ion channel of *N*-methyl-D-Aspartate (NMDA) receptors [4].

Perhaps the dopamine hypothesis would do best today if it were understood in terms of a dysregulation rather than overt hyperdopaminergia, as originally proposed. This dysregulation may arise within the dopaminergic neuron itself or in adjacent neuronal circuitries.

Our own efforts to widen the perspective started about 8 years ago, when we tried to find an explanation for the paradox that antipsychotic agents, which apparently exert powerful actions on the cerebral cortex, have as their main targets dopamine D_2 receptors which are very sparse in the human cerebral cortex. There is, of course, the possibility that the cortical D_2 receptors are nevertheless sufficiently abundant to be the relevant targets for antipsychotic action – after all, the brain is not a democracy. Alternatively, antipsychotic action may be linked to some other receptors, such as the D_4 receptors, even if this latter alternative seems less likely at present. In any event we felt tempted to try to develop a hypothetical model that might serve to explain how subcortically located dopamine receptors could exert a profound effect on cortical functions, assuming that the antipsychotic agents had their predominant action in brain regions where the dopamine receptors are most abundant, that is, in the basal ganglia, and that the actions on the cortex were thus largely indirect.

Based on available neuroanatomical evidence [5–7], we then came up with a model which, although simplistic, might serve as a starting point [8]. We postulated that the striatal complexes, comprising the dorsal and ventral striatum and the corresponding dorsal and ventral pallidum, exert a predominantly inhibitory function on the thalamus, leading to a reduced transmission of sensory information to the cerebral cortex as well as a concomitant reduction of arousal. As is generally recognized, arousal is controlled by the ascending reticular formation, which operates in close linkage to the sensory input. We assume that dopamine is predominantly inhibitory on striatal neurons, and thus an increased dopaminergic tone should counteract the inhibitory impact of the striatal complexes on the thalamus and, consequently, enhance the transmission of sensory information to the cortex and raise the level of arousal. If the transmission through the thalamus becomes excessive, the integrative capacity of the cortex may break down, and confusion or psychosis will ensue.

It may be appropriate on this occasion to pay tribute to the father of clozapine at the preclinical level, that is, Günther Stille. The only time I can remember having met him was at the above-mentioned meeting in Stockholm in 1974. He gave a paper at this meeting dealing with the neurophysiological correlates to antipsychotic drug effects [9]. I have to confess that I did not understand much of it at that time. However, I have read it once again, and I now find it a lot more interesting. In fact his conclusions are similar to the suggestions put forward above. In Stille's electrophysiological studies the striatum shows up as an inhibitory structure within the strio-pallido-thalamo-cortical system. Electrical stimulation of caudate neurons by short series of 40–200 Hz was found to lower the amplitude of the cortical potentials evoked by afferent sensory stimuli. Neuroleptics were found to increase the electrical activity of caudate neurons and would thus presumably also lower the amplitude of the cortical potentials evoked by afferent sensory stimuli, even though this assumption was not supported by experimental data.

Stille also emphasized the antagonism between the striatum and the ascending reticular formation with respect to arousal and gating. Neuroleptics acted on the reticular formation in an inhibitory fashion. Some neuroleptic drugs, for example haloperidol, had their predominating action on the striatum, which would predict extrapyramidal side effects (EPS), whereas others, with clozapine as the most striking example, acted preferentially on the reticular formation, which in his opinion would account for its much lower EPS liability.

So far, Stille's observations seemed reasonably straightforward, but he pointed out that, paradoxically, neuroleptics had also been found to *increase* the amplitude of the evoked response in the cortex. He proposed an interesting hypothetical explanation for this contradiction, based on some observations indicating that tonic and phasic stimulation of the caudate could lead to opposite effects on cortical evoked responses. The inhibitory effect of the caudate would be induced by stimulating it tonically, whereas phasic stimulation would facilitate the evoked responses. This is interesting in view of more recent neuroanatomical and pharmacological findings to be discussed next, which support such a dual function of the striatum. I think it is fair to say today that Stille was ahead of his time.

At that time it was not known that the dopaminergic inhibitory influence on the striatum is counterbalanced by a powerful glutamatergic excitatory input from all parts of the cortex as well as from the thalamus. A deficient glutamatergic tone should lead to a similar condition as an elevated dopaminergic tone, i.e., excessive transmission of sensory information and hyperarousal, ultimately leading to confusion or psychosis. On the other hand, a reduced dopaminergic tone induced, e.g., by neuroleptic agents, might lead to glutamatergic predominance, increased striatal activity, and reduced sensory input reaching the cortex, and thus to a similar situation as that induced by tonic electrical stimulation of the striatum.

The striatum is generally believed to regulate both motility and mental functions; the dorsal striatum is often assumed to be involved in motor functions, whereas the ventral striatum might rather serve to control mental functions. However, this distinction may not be as sharp as is often assumed. For example, rostral parts of the dorsal striatum may be important for cognitive functions. Their strong projections from the frontal lobes speak in favor of this theory [10].

When we speak of the cerebral cortex in this context we refer to the cortex in a wide sense – comprising, for example, the prefrontal cortex, the gyrus cinguli, the hippocampus, and so forth. Probably some parts of the cortex are more important than others in the regulation of the functions discussed here, and different authors emphasize the importance of certain regions, such as the prefrontal cortex or the hippocampus.

Dopamine-Glutamate Interactions

When dopaminergic function is reduced, this will, as already mentioned, lead to inhibition of motility and mental activity. A simple way to test the predictive value of the present model would be to induce a drastic state of hypodopaminergia, leading to immobility, and then to inhibit the corticostriatal glutamatergic function. If this model is valid, mobility should then be restored despite the absence of dopamine. We did this experiment in 1989, and it came out in the predicted way [11]. In this experiment we depleted mice of dopamine by means of reserpine in combination with alpha-methyltyrosine. The immobility thus induced was dramatically reversed by systemic treatment with the NMDA receptor antagonist MK-801. Later the same effect was induced by local treatment with NMDA receptor antagonists, e.g. AP-5 [12]. The local treatment actually gave more striking results because the pattern of the movements thus restored was more normal than after systemic treatment. In the latter case but not in the former, ataxia and inability to switch motor program were observed.

The main significance of these experiments is that they show that the glutamatergic system can control motility and arousal independently of dopamine and in fact in the complete absence of dopamine. To prove this, it was necessary to use the treatment strategy involving both reserpine and alpha-methyltyrosine, because there is hardly any known alternative treatment where a role of dopamine can be completely ruled out. In our experiments we could confirm this by demonstrating that the motility restored by means of antiglutamatergic agents could not be blocked by dopamine-receptor blocking agents.

The issue of dopamine-glutamate interaction needs, however, some further elaboration. Even though glutamate can control psychomotor activity independently of dopamine, a powerful interaction between dopamine and glutamate can be demonstrated. Thus, when subthreshold doses of apomorphine, a mixed D_1/D_2 agonist, and MK-801, a noncompetitive NMDA receptor antagonist, are combined, a strong potentiation occurs, showing up as motility in monoamine-depleted mice [13–16]. Since no endogenous dopamine is available in these experiments, the interaction between the two neurotransmitters must be assumed to occur postsynaptically, presumably on striatal GABAergic projection neurons. That this interaction also occurs in mice not depleted of monoamines is supported by the fact that psychomotor stimulation can be induced by a lower dose of MK-801 in normal than in monoamine-depleted mice and that this effect can be antagonized by dopamine receptor antagonists in mice with intact monoaminergic systems, in contrast to monoamine-depleted mice. Thus MK-801 in a lower dose range seems to stimulate motility at least partly by increasing the sensitivity to endogenous dopamine. Originally it was proposed that MK-801 could stimulate motility by increasing the release of monoamines [17]. However, the available data on this issue are not conclusive. Whereas some authors report an increased release of dopamine by MK-801 treatment in microdialysis experiments, others have failed to observe this effect. In the case of competitive NMDA receptor antagonists, stimulation of motility has been demonstrated concomitantly with evidence of an unchanged or even *decreased* dopamine release. Interestingly, competitive NMDA antagonists, in contrast to noncompetitive antagonists, require higher doses to stimulate motility in normal mice, as compared to monoamine-depleted mice (review and discussion in [18]).

Dual Function of Striatal Glutamate

The data discussed so far indicate the existence of a powerful antagonism between dopamine and glutamate in the striatum. However, as mentioned, the picture is more complicated, judging by various pieces of evidence. The striatum appears to control the thalamus by both "direct" and "indirect" pathways, containing chains of two and three GABAergic neurons, respectively [19, 20] (Fig. 1). Since both pathways are controlled by corticostriatal glutamatergic neurons, it follows that these neurons should function in opposite directions. Those controlling the indirect pathways should be inhibitory and those controlling the direct pathways, stimulating at the thalamic level. This contention is supported by the following pharmacological evidence.

The interaction between dopamine and glutamate at the postsynaptic striatal level seems to depend to some degree on the extent to which D_1 and D_2 receptors are involved. The psychomotor stimulation induced by NMDA receptor antagonists in combination with a dopamine D_1 agonist provides evidence of potentiation, wthereas the combination with a dopamine D_2 agonist indicates an antagonistic interaction. However, the outcome of these combined treatments is partly dependent on the baseline activity level [13–16]. It is tempting to suggest that the differential interaction between glutamate and dopamine D_1 and D_2 receptors may be related to indirect and direct pathways, respectively, although direct support for this speculation is not available [21].

An even more striking demonstration of the dual function of striatal glutamate on behavior is obtained by local unilateral administration of an NMDA receptor antagonist such as AP-5 in the nucleus accumbens. In rats with an intact monoaminergic system, this treatment results in ipsilateral rotation, whereas in monoamine-depleted rats the same treatment causes contralateral rotation. If the latter animals are treated systemically with a dopamine D_2 receptor agonist the rotation switches from contralateral to ipsilateral. It would thus appear that glutamate serves a dual function and that the direction of the function depends on the D_2-dopaminergic tone [22].

In conclusion, a dual function of the striatum with respect to the control of the thalamic filter is supported by the electrophysiologic data of Stille [9] as well as by neuroanatomical and pharmacological observations. Maybe this will provide more

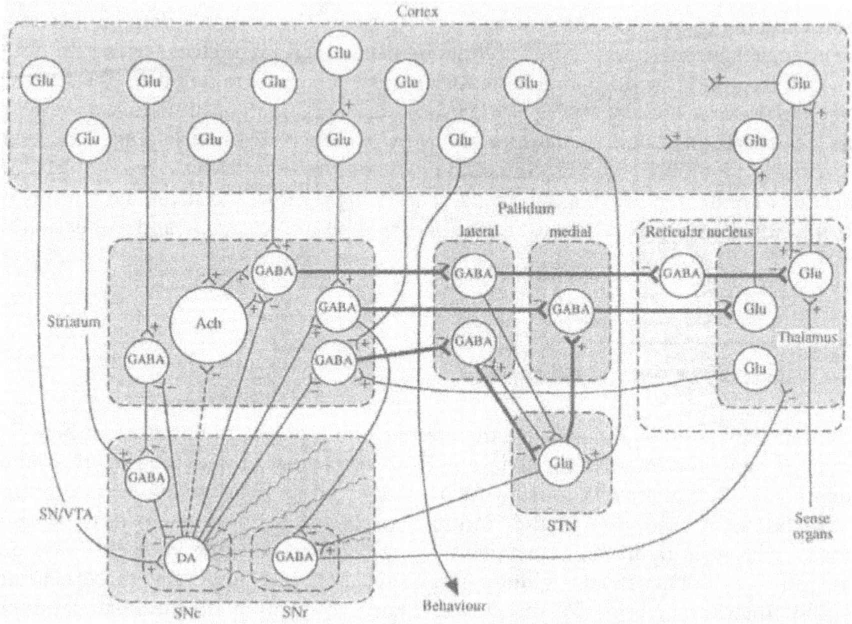

Fig. 1. Neurocircuitries of the basal ganglia. The pathways drawn with *thick lines* indicate some connections between the striatum and the thalamus which are discussed in some detail in this chapter. The *top* and *bottom* pathways drawn with thick lines each contain three GABAergic neurons and are referred to as "indirect" pathways. The pathway in between contains two GABAergic neurons and is referred to as "direct". *SN*, substantia nigra; *VTA*, ventral tegmental area; *STN*, subthalamic nucleus; *Glu*, glutamate; *Ach*, acetylcholine; *DA*, dopamine; *SNc*, Substantia nigra pars compacta; *SNr*, Substantia nigra pars reticula (Modified from [26])

profound insights into the function of the striatum. Stille proposed that a tonic stimulation of striatal neurons would induce an inhibitory influence on the thalamus, whereas a phasic stimulation would be facilitating. In this context it is interesting that the direct pathway has been proposed to be operating mainly by phasic activity [20], whereas the indirect pathway is driven by tonic stimulation. A possible interpretation could be that the indirect pathway, by means of tonic activity, serves to suppress the passage of sensory "background noise" through the thalamus to the cortex, and to promote habituation, whereas the tonic activity of the direct pathway would serve to amplify the passage of novel, significant information. It may be speculated that the sensory input initially reaching the cortex is first scanned against stored information and thus evaluated with respect to novelty and significance. The cortex will then send messages to the striatum via the glutamatergic pathways, leading to suppression of trivial information through the indirect pathways and amplification of the significant input through the direct pathways. A defect in the indirect pathway might lead to positive symptoms and a defect in the direct pathway to negative symptoms.

The interaction between dopamine and glutamate is further complicated by the fact that NMDA receptor antagonists can influence the firing pattern of dopaminergic neurons [23]. The relative importance of the interactions between dopamine and glutamate at these various levels cannot be assessed at present. It may vary depending on the location within the dopaminergic system, the baseline activity, and a variety of experimental conditions. However, generally speaking, the level of dopaminergic tone may determine the balance between the facilitating and inhibitory impact of the striatum on the thalamus.

Role of Other Neurotransmitters in Psychotogenesis

Continued work along these lines has demonstrated a broad spectrum of interactions between dopamine, glutamate, noradrenaline, serotonin, and acetylcholine with respect to psychomotor activity. Since these interactions can also occur in monoamine-depleted mice it seems clear that not only glutamate but also noradrenaline, serotonin, and acetylcholine can influence psychomotor activity by mechanisms that do not involve variations in dopaminergic tone but must be assumed to occur postsynaptically in relation to the dopaminergic neurons. However, just as in the case of dopamine-glutamate interactions, there is evidence that both noradrenergic and serotonergic influences can be dramatically enhanced by reduction of glutamatergic tone. Thus the interactions between a variety of neurotransmitters should be taken into account in considerations related to psychotogenesis [24–34].

Some recent data from our laboratory illustrate the interaction of serotonin and 5-HT_2 receptors with other systems controlling psychomotor activity. The stimulant action of LSD is strongly potentiated by MK-801 in monoamine-depleted mice, and this effect can be blocked by the potent and selective 5-HT_{2A} receptor antagonist MDL 100,907. We thus have another example here of the capacity of glutamate to prevent psychomotor hyperactivity. In mice with an intact monoaminergic system the psychostimulant action of MK-801 can be antagonized by MDL 100,907. Insofar as the MK-801-treated mouse can serve as a psychosis model, we can thus conclude that there is room not only for dopaminergic antagonists but also for 5-HT_2 receptor antagonists as therapeutic candidates. In fact, the psychostimulant action of atropine can also be antagonized by MDL 100,907 (unpublished data of this laboratory).

From the point of view of psychotogenesis, these observations are interesting, given the fact that all the neurotransmitters mentioned previously have been shown to induce or alleviate psychosis. Given these close interactions, none of these neurotransmitters can be disregarded when discussing the etiology or pathogenesis of schizophrenia or other psychotic conditions. Figure 2 shows a scheme with indications of possible cortical and subcortical sites of action of various psychotomimetic agents. Needless to say, this scheme is speculative and does not claim to be in any way comprehensive. Rather it is meant to serve as a starting point for testing various hypotheses of psychotogenic mechanisms.

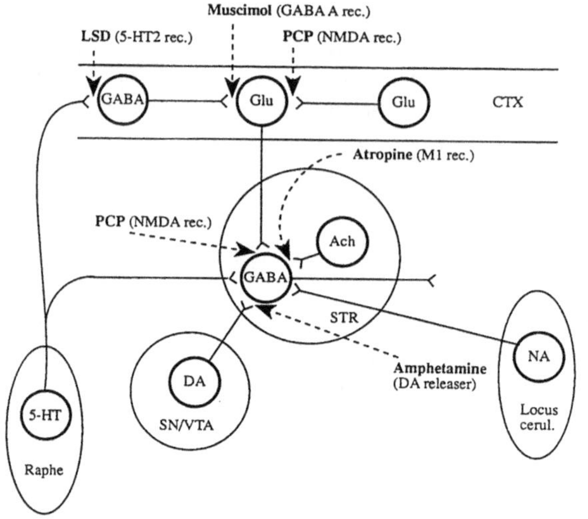

Fig. 2. Schematic diagram illustrating potential psychotogenic pathways and sites of action of psychotogenic and antipsychotic agents. Amphetamine and phencyclidine (PCP) are thought to be psychotogenic by acting at least partly on striatal dompamine (*DA*) release and *N*-methyl-D-aspartate (NMDA) receptors, respectively, in the (limbic) striatum, although other sites may contribute. For example, PCP may act by blocking cortical NMDA receptors as well, e.g., in the hipoqcampus, as indicated in this figure, leading to reduced tone in corticostriatal glutamatergic pathways. The 5-HT_2 agonist LSD may act by stimulating cortical GABAergic interneurons, thereby reducing corticostriatal glutamatergic tone [37]. LSD also seems to act on neurons in the striatum. The GABA A receptor agonist muscimol, which also appears to be psychotogenic [38], may likewise act by reducing corticostriatal glutamatergic tone. Anticholinergic agents appear to act by blocking predominantly muscarinic M_1 receptors. *CTX*, cortex; *STR*, striatum; *Locus cerul.*, locus caeruleus; *NA*, noradrenaline.

From the point of view of drug development, the behavioral model presented there is versatile, in that it permits demonstration of interactions with virtually all the major endogenous players in psychotogenesis at pre- as well as postsynaptic levels. I now wish to turn to some work that has prompted us to develop a biochemical psychosis model, which in our opinion will serve as an important supplement to the behavioral models.

Postmortem Studies Leading to a Tentative Biochemical Model of Schizophrenia

This work starts out from some postmortem studies that we have performed on brains from schizophrenic patients. I will limit myself here to one of these studies. Here we have analyzed several brain regions with regard to monoaminergic indices, that is, the levels of dopamine, noradrenaline, and serotonin as well as some of their precursors and metabolites. Using conventional univariate statistics we were unable to detect any striking differences between controls and schizophrenics, treated as a single group. However, when multivariate statistics were applied, the outcome was different [35]. The schizophrenics showed an almost complete separation from the controls but showed up in two different groups located on either side of the controls (Figure 3). Moreover, the two schizophrenic subgroups differed in terms of diagnostic categories, in that one of them consisted of paranoid and the other of nonparanoid schizophrenics. When applying univariate statistics on the two subgroups we found

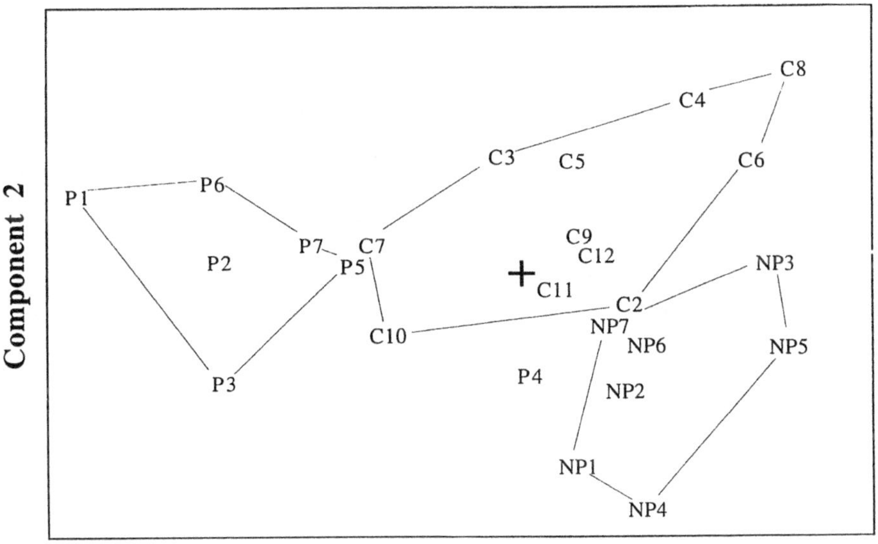

Fig. 3. Principal least squares discriminant analysis (PLSDA) of monoaminergic indices in several brain regions of chronic schizophrenic patients and age-matched controls. The monoaminergic indices measured were dopamine, 3-methoxy-tyramine, serotonin, 5-hydroxytryptophan, 5-hydroxyindoleacetic acid, noradrenaline, normetanephrine, tyrosine, and tryptophan. *C*, controls; *P*, paranoid schizophrenics; *NP*, "non-paranoid" schizophrenics. (From [35])

that several biochemical variables differed significantly from the controls, and that in many cases they differed in opposite directions for the two diagnostic subgroups. It was of course also possible to treat either subgroup in a multivariate analysis and compare it with the controls. We now found that the biochemical pattern showing up in the paranoid subgroup was similar to that found in rats treated with the glutamatergic antagonist MK-801. This similarity invites the speculation that glutamatergic deficiency may be an important factor in paranoid schizophrenia.

To illustrate the potential usefulness of this model we have compared the action of haloperidol and MDL 100,907 in regard to their ability to normalize the biochemical aberrations induced by MK-801. The 5-HT_{2A} antagonist was found to bring about a fairly satisfactory normalization, whereas haloperidol had a more complex action on the biochemical pattern.

Therapeutic Implications

One of the most striking features emerging from the present animal studies is the evidence for a strong impact of corticofugal glutamatergic pathways on the function of a variety of subcortical systems, which depend for their function on dopaminergic, noradrenergic, serotonergic, cholinergic, and GABAergic neurotransmitters. In the case of the three first-mentioned monoaminergic systems, glutamate appears to have a predominantly inhibitory influence, even though, at least in the case of D_2 mediated dopaminergic function, glutamate and dopamine may also act in concert. In the case of cholinergic mechanisms, glutamate seems to have a mainly enhancing influence. As a consequence of these various influences it would appear that, for example, a glutamatergic deficiency involving corticofugal pathways should have a pronounced impact on a variety of subcortical systems. In several cases the consequence would be a disinhibition of these systems. Such disinhibition might well contribute to the psychotic symptoms observed, for example, in schizophrenia. If, in addition, a glutamatergic deficiency also exists in intracortical association systems this might contribute to certain aspects of the symptomatology, such as cognitive defect, ambivalence, and part of the negative symptomatology.

Another possible mechanism underlying negative symptoms could be related to insufficient glutamatergic stimulation of the positive feedback loops described earlier in this review.

At present there does not seem to be any convincing, well-established evidence in favor of a glutamatergic deficiency in schizophrenia. However, this does not speak very strongly against "the glutamate hypothesis of schizophrenia" [36], taking into account the methodological problems involved in these kinds of studies. Thus it appears warranted to examine the possibility of manipulating glutamatergic functions in schizophrenia in order to attain relief of the symptomatology. In this context the use of agonists acting on one of the glutamatergic receptors would seem especially appropriate. However, in view of the ubiquitous distribution of glutamatergic pathways in the brain and their involvement in a variety of functions, such as control of convulsion threshold and leaming, as well as the risk of excitotoxicity, this approach will probably turn out to be difficult. Possibly the use of partial agonists, the manipulation of allosteric sites on the glutamatergic receptors, or the use of subtype-specific agonists, yet to be discovered, may ultimately turn out successfully.

Even if glutamatergic deficiency may be an important pathogenetic factor in schizophrenia, therapeutic manipulation of the other systems involved in psychotogenesis may still have a lot to offer. This is true, for example, of 5-HT_2 receptor antagonists; trials with such agents to be expected in the near future are thus eagerly awaited. Moreover, several other transmitter systems remain to be more thoroughly explored, and this is no less true of the dopaminergic system. The various receptor subtypes recently discovered certainly need further exploration, and even the classical D_1 and D_2 subtypes, which are quantitatively dominating, have not yet been sufficiently examined. This is particularly true of the D_2 subtype, whose importance for psychotogenesis has been most convincingly demonstrated. A strategy aiming to stabilize rather than inhibit dopaminergic function would appear especially attractive.

Drugs which combine two or more of the mechanisms indicated above may of course possess a considerable therapeutic potential. Clozapine is an important representative of this type of agent, and several other drugs with multiple sites of action are now being or have already been introduced in the treatment of psychosis, e.g., risperidone, olanzapine, seroquel, and sertindole.

The intense research efforts now ongoing in the area of schizophrenia, with new insights emerging from basic as well as clinical research, call for some optimism. After a long period of relative stagnation in the therapy of schizophrenia we can expect some exciting developments during the next 5 to 10 years.

References

1. Deniker P (1983) Discovery of the clinical use of neuroleptics. In: Parnham MJ, Bruinvels J (eds) Psycho- and neuropharmacology. Elsevier, Amsterdam, pp 163–180 (Discoveries in pharmacology, vol 1)
2. Hippius H (1976) On the relation between antipsychotic and extrapyramidal effects of psychoactive drugs. In: Sedvall G, Uvnäs B, Zotterman Y (eds) Antipsychotic drugs: pharmacodynamics and pharmacokinetics. Pergamon, Oxford, pp 437–446
3. Domino E, Luby ED (1973) Abnormal mental states induced by phencyclidine as a model of schizophrenia. In: Cole JO, Freedman AM, Friedhoff AJ (eds) Psychopathology and psychopharmacology. Johns Hopkins University Press, Baltimore, pp 37–50
4. Lodge D, Aran JA, Church J, Davies SN, Martin D, Zeman S (1987) Excitatory amino acids and phencyclidine drugs. In: Hicks TP, Lodge D, McLennan H (eds) Excitatory amino acid transmission. Liss, New York, pp 83–90
5. Heimer L, Alheid GF, Zaborszky L (1985) Basal ganglia. In: Paxinos G (ed) Forebrain and midbrain. Academic, New York, pp 37–86 (The rat nervous system, vol 1)
6. Heimer L, de Olmos J, Alheid GF, Zaborszky L (1991) "Perestroika" in the basal forebrain: opening the border between neurology and psychiatry. Prog Brain Res 87: 109–165
7. Alheid G, Heimer L, Switzer RC (1990) The basal ganglia. In: Paxinos G (ed) The human nervous system. Academic, San Diego, pp 483–582
8. Carlsson A (1988) The current status of the dopamine hypothesis of schizophrenia. With commentaries and author's reply. Neuropsychopharmacology 1: 179–203
9. Stille G (1976) Neurophysiological correlates to antipsychotic effects of drugs. In: Sedvall G, Uvnäs B, Zotterman Y (eds) Antipsychotic Drugs: pharmacodynamics and pharmacokinetics. Pergamon, Oxford, pp 51–62
10. Goldman-Rakic PS, Selemon LD (1986) Topography of corticostriatal projections in nonhuman primates and implications for functional parcellation of the neostriatum. In: Jones EG, Peters A (eds) Cerebral cortex, vol 5. Plenum, New York, pp 447–466
11. Carlsson M, Carlsson A (1989) The NMDA antagonist MK-801 causes marked locomotor stimulation in monoamine-depleted mice. J Neural Transm 75: 221–226
12. Svensson A, Carlsson ML (1992) Injection of the competitive NMDA receptor antagonist AP-5 into the nucleus accumbens of monoamine-depleted mice induces pronounced locomotor stimulation. Neuropharmacology 31: 513–518
13. Svensson A, Carlsson A, Carlsson ML (1992) Differential locomotor interactions between dopamine D_1/D_2 receptor agonists and the NMDA antagonist dizocilpine in monoamine-depleted mice. J Neural Transm Gen Sect 90: 199–217
14. Starr MS, Starr BS (1993). Glutamate antagonists modify the motor stimulant actions of D_1 and D_2 agonists in reserpine-treated mice in complex ways that are not predictive of their interactions with the mixed D1/D2 agonist apomorphine. J Neural Transm Park Dis Dement Sect 6: 215–226
15. Starr MS, Starr BS (1993) Facilitation of dopamine D1 receptor – but not dopamine D_1/D_2 receptor-dependent locomotion by glutamate antagonists in the reserpine-treated mouse. Eur J Pharmacol 250: 239–246
16. Morelli M, Di Chiara G (1990) MK-801 potentiates dopaminergic D_1 but reduces D_2 responses in the 6-hydroxydopamine model of Parkinson's disease. Eur J Pharmacol 182: 611–612

17. Clineschmidt BV, Martin GE, Bunting PR, Papp NL (1982) Central sympathomimetic activity of (+)-5-methyl-10,11-dihydro(a,d)cyclo-hepten-5,10-imine (MK-801), a substance with potent anticonvulsant, central sympathomimetic and apparent anxiolytic properties. Drug Dev Res 2: 135–145
18. Carlsson ML (1993) Are the disparate pharmacological profiles of competitive and uncompetitive NMDA antagonists due to different baseline activities of distinct glutamatergic pathways? (Hypothesis). J Neural Transm Gen Sect 9: 1–10
19. Penney JB, Young AB (1986) Striatal inhomogeneities and basal ganglia function. Mov Disord 1: 3–15
20. Alexander GE, Crutcher MD (1990) Functional architecture of basal ganglia circuits: neural substrates of parallel processing. Trends Neurosci 13: 266–271
21. Gerfen CR, Engber TM, Mahan LC et al. (1990) D_1 and D_2 dopamine receptor-regulated gene expression of striatonigral and striatopallidal neurons. Science 250: 1429–1432
22. Svensson A, Carlsson ML, Carlsson A (1992) Interaction between glutamatergic and dopaminergic tone in the nucleus accumbens of mice: evidence for a dual glutamatergic function with respect to psychomotor control. J Neural Transm Gen Sect 88: 235–240
23. Svensson TH (1995) Mode of action of atypical neuroleptics in relation to the phencyclidine model of schizophrenia: role of 5-HT_2 receptor and α_1-adrenoceptor antagonism. J Clin Psychopharmacol 15 Suppl 1: 11S–18S
24. Carlsson M, Carlsson A (1989) Marked locomotor stimulation in monoamine-depleted mice following treatment with atropine in combination with clonidine. J Neural Transm Park Dis Dement Sect 1: 317–322
25. Carlsson M, Carlsson A (1989) Dramatic synergism between MK-801 and clonidine with respect to locomotor stimulatory effect in monoamine-depleted mice. J Neural Transm Gen Sect 77: 65–71
26. Carlsson M, Carlsson A (1990) Interactions between glutamatergic and mono-aminergic systems within the basal ganglia – implications for schizophrenia and Parkinson's disease. Trends Neurosci 13: 272–276
27. Carlsson M, Carlsson A (1990) Schizophrenia: a subcortical neurotransmitter imbalance syndrome? Schizophr Bull 16: 425–432
28. Carlsson M, Svensson A (1990) Interfering with glutamatergic neurotransmission by means of NMDA antagonist administration discloses the locomotor stimulatory potential of other transmitter systems. Pharmacol Biochem Behav 3: 45–50
29. Carlsson M, Svensson A (1990) The non-competitive NMDA antagonists MK-801 and PCP, as well as the competitive NMDA antagonist SDZ EAA494 (D-CPPene), interact synergistically with clonidine to promote locomotion in monoamine-depleted mice. Life Sci 47: 1729–1736
30. Carlsson M, Svensson A, Carlsson A (1991) Synergistic interactions between muscarinic antagonists and NMDA antagonists with respect to locomotor stimulatory effects in monoamine-depleted mice. Naunyn Schmiedebergs Arch Pharmacol 343: 568–573
31. Carlsson ML, Engberg G, Carlsson A (1994) Effects of D-cycloserine and (+)-HA-966 on the locomotor stimulation induced by NMDA antagonists and clonidine in monoamine-depleted mice. J Neural Transm Gen Sect 95: 223–233
32. Svensson A, Carlsson ML (1995) The muscarine antagonist methscopolamine and the NMDA antagonist AP-5 injected unilaterally into the nucleus accumbens cause mice to rotate in opposite directiones. J Neural Transm Gen Sect (in press)
33. Svensson A, Carlsson ML, Carlsson A (1994) Glutamatergic neurons projecting to the nucleus accumbens can affect motor functions in opposite directions depending on the dopaminergic tone. Prog Neuro psychopharmacol Biol Psychiatry 18: 1203–1218
34. Svensson A, Carlsson ML, Carlsson A (1995) Crucial role of the accumbens nucleus in the neurotransmitter interactions regulating motor control in mice. J Neural Trans Gen Sect (in press)
35. Hansson LO, Waters N, Winblad B, Gottfries C-G, Carlsson A (1994) Evidence for biochemical heterogeneity in schizophrenia: a multivariante study of monoaminergic indices in human post-mortem brain tissue. J Neural Transm Gen Sect 98: 217–235
36. Kornhuber HH, Kornhuber J, Kim JS, Kornhuber ME (1984) Zur biochemischen Theorie der Schizophrenie. Nervenarzt 55: 602–606
37. Gellman RL, Aghajanian GK (1991) IPSPs in pyramidal cells in piriform cortex evoked by monoamine excitation of interneurons demonstrate a convergence of inputs. Soc Neurosci Abstr 17: 1: 989
38. Tamminga CA, Crayton JC, Chase TN (1978) Muscimol: GABA agonist therapy in schizophrenia. Am J Psychiatry 135: 746–748

The Etiology of Affective Illness

F. K. Goodwin

The introduction of effective psychopharmacological drugs four decades ago sparked a revolution that has, over time, reshaped scientific and popular concepts of mental illness. Like all revolutionary periods, the era blazed with activity, as investigators conducted studies into the neurobiological mechanisms that might explain the powerful, specific effects of the new drugs. Recurrent major affective illness – manic depressive illness in classical Kraepelin terms – quickly became the clinical mainstay for such research, a model for biological studies on other major mental illness. More homogeneous than nonrecurrent unipolar depression or schizophrenia, manic depressive illness attracted scientific attention for other reasons as well: Its genetic diathesis (reviewed by Gershon in this volume) was clear to many clinicians treating the illness; its cyclic nature – particularly the bipolar subtype – gave investigators the opportunity to study the transition phases and to separate the traits intrinsic to the illness from the state changes that accompany being ill; and finally, lithium's effects on both poles of the bipolar subtype presented an irresistible scientific challenge.

Today our understanding of the neurobiology of severe mental illness is once again undergoing a transformation, this time sparked by the rapid maturation of the neurosciences over the past few years. Molecular and cellular neuroscience reveals increasingly complex mechanisms at the most fundamental level of biological organization. Such insights may finally clarify the mechanisms of action of psychoactive medications, a development that should lead rapidly to more specific pharmacological agents. Improved imaging techniques provide a clinical approach to the critical questions about how brain systems interact in producing complex behavior. These clinical studies are beginning to confirm findings from animal research on the extensive integration of information flow within the brain and the ways in which responses to external stimuli are remarkably regulated toward homeostasis. Characterizing these pathways may lead to better understanding of the pathogenesis of mental illness.

Developments in molecular genetics could also alter central assumptions about severe mental illness. Many of us matured scientifically during the era when genetic epidemiology was demonstrating once and for all that severe mental illness has a substantial heritable component. Implicit in most conceptual models of these illness is the notion of a genetic diathesis activated by environmental stressors to produce the onset of illness. This so-called diathesis-stress model is being refined as the search for the molecular genetic basis of mental illness suggests complex patterns of inheritance. We may, for example, come to speak of "vulnerabilities", a constellation of genetic traits on the diathesis end of the equation. Experience in other relatively common diseases, such as Alzheimer's and breast cancer, suggests heterogeneous diatheses; those forms with the earliest onset and most virulent course may be the most heritable and – if that genetic component can be identified – may yield clues to the pathogenesis of all forms. Compared with other severe mental illnesses, however, manic-depressive illness – particularly in its bipolar subtye – is relatively homogeneous and thus is the focus of much of this pioneering work.

In this chapter I point out some of the recent findings on the neurobiology of manic-depressive illness and discuss them in the context of previous conceptions. I begin by reviewing the evolution of research on the neurobiology of manic-depressive illness, followed by a few recent developments in identifiying vulnerability markers and in elucidating the biology of recurrence – two lines of research that seem to hold particular promise in disentangling pathophysiology.

Classically, manic-depressive illness comprised all severe forms of affective illness. Besides the tendency to recur, severe unipolar illness shares other characteristics with bipolar disorder (e.g., prophylactic response to lithium). As we have argued elsewhere (Goodwin and Jamison 1990), separating bipolar and unipolar disorders in formal diagnostic systems prejudges the relationship between them, giving priority to polarity and neglecting the cyclicity common to both forms. Important questions are thus never asked: For example, since bipolar illness is more recurrent, are reported differences with unipolar illness a function of greater cyclicity or are they simply related to a history of mania?

Lability, variability, and fluctuation tend to characterize most clinical features of manic-depressive illness, between patients and within the same patient from one episode to the next. Besides the episodic nature of the illness, these fluctuations in symptoms, course, severity, and treatment response may provide the single most important clue to pathophysiology. They suggest a profound dysregulation in normal homeostatic processes, one that may involve central pacemakers designed to keep physiological systems synchronized. That possibility is one of many areas now being explored in neurobiological studies of manic-depressive illness.

Once the effectiveness of the antidepressants and lithium became obvious, investigators began using the drug's action as a bridge to understanding pathophysiological processes. The amine hypotheses were formulated by linking the effects of drugs on brain amine systems in animals to their clinical effects on the depressed (or manic) state. The early studies of acute presynaptic effects of drugs eventually gave way to an emphasis on longer term receptor adaptation both pre- and postsynaptically. But the focus continues to change. In my view, an ideal biological hypothesis about major affective illness must be able to account for the two most fundamental characteristics of the illness – genetic vulnerability and recurrence. Here I review some interesting advances that get us closer to that ideal.

The great majority of direct biological studies of patients has focused on changes that accompany the illness state. Most of these essentially cross-sectional studies clinically evaluate the amine hypotheses derived from animal pharmacology. State-independent biological abnormalities, the focus of clinical genetic studies, are often identified as predisposing traits but in fact are derived from studies of recovered patients. A vulnerability marker, by contrast, must be identified in subjects before they become depressed. To do this, longitudinal studies are needed in populations at risk (for now, the first-degree relatives of depressed patients).

None of the putative markers studied to date (e.g. enzymes involved in amine metabolism) has as yet fulfilled the requirements of an illness marker: that it covary with the illness in pedigrees. Although somewhat limited for ethical reasons, challenge paradigms are promising; one such type of study uses stress activation in investigations of the learned helplessness paradigm (Breier et al. 1987).

A further complication to interpreting state-trait difference has become apparent as evidence for homeostatic processes in the brain accumulates. Post and Weiss (1992) argue that some characteristic physiological changes in affective illness may represent the body's drive toward homeostasis. Thus, the failure of thyroid-releasing hormone and dexamethasone suppression to return to normal after an affective episode, which has been associated with a vulnerability to relapse (Gurguis et al 1990), may be directly related to the pathological process. Alternatively, these physiological responses could represent adaptations compensating for some other primary pathological process. Underscoring this point, McEwen et al. (1992) demonstrate that adrenal steroids serve an adaptive and protective function, mediating the influence of environmental stress on brain structure, chemistry, and activity through alterations in gene expression and changes in cell membranes. But the well-recognized immunosuppression and destruction of hippocampal neurons characterize another phase of their action. These regulatory and counterregulatory effects emphasize that the homeostatic processes integrating brain functioning occur in concert with other processes, over time.

Recent attempts to identify characteristics of major affective illness that distinguish it from other psychopathology suggest that investigators have become increasingly sensitive to trait-state issues, a promising development that should speed progress in the field. Interactions between neurotransmitter, neuroendocrine, and other systems are more often the focus of study as the resolution of imaging techniques and other new technology continues to improve. For example, a considerable body of evidence has begun to clarify how the sympathetic nervous system and glucocorticoids maintain homeostasis in the serotonin system during stress (Chaouloff 1993). This same body of work may, incidentally, hold a clue to the greater vulnerability of women to depressive illness. At a finer level of organization, other work is focusing on intracellular processes, the second-messenger systems that may be the endpoint of drug action. Much of this research examines changes in gene expression that may partly account for changes in disease course and treatment response.

Like other pathophysiological investigations of manic-depressive illness, neuropathological and imaging studies must be interpreted in the context of alterations accompanying the state of illness. Computed tomography (CT) and magnetic resonance imaging (MRI) studies have shown structural brain abnormalities, and some suggest these alterations are greater in bipolar than in unipolar patients. Although not as extensively studied as schizophrenia, bipolar illness has, in some studies, been accompanied by the ventricular enlargement or increased ventricular/brain ratios commonly found in schizophrenia. Andreasen et al. (1990), for example, found that male bipolar patients had significantly larger ventricles on a CT scan than unipolar depressed patients and normal subjects. The ventricular enlargement appeared to be independent of age (as it is in schizophrenia), and did not correlate with treatment response, past substance abuse, a history of electroconvulsive therapy, or cognitive impairment. Whether the observed anomalies are state or trait markers remains unclear. Also unclear is whether the changes represent neurodevelopmental anomalies or a degenerative process related to repeated episodes, as suggested by Altshuler (1993). Arguing against a degenerative process are the results of a study by Woods et al. (1990), who found evidence of progressive enlargement in ventricular size over 2 1/2 years in patients with schizophrenia but not in patients with bipolar illness. In a recent study of first-episode manic patients, Strakowski et al. (1993) found significantly larger third ventricles in bipolar patients than in normal subjects. This finding could mean that the ventricular changes predated the first appearance of mania, possibly constituting a trait marker. But this and other imaging studies should be interpreted in light of evidence that the hypercortisolemia characterstics of depression and severe mania may in itself lead to changes in the extracellular fluid pool, which could show up as ventricular enlargement. Strakowski et al. (1993) also report abnormal gray/white matter distribution in patients going through a first episode of mania, particularly women. Although preliminary and possibly an artifact of physical movement, this finding is interesting in light of recent reports of increased rates of signal hyperintensity in bipolar patients (e.g., Dupont et al. 1987; Swayze et al. 1992a).

Swayze et al. (1992b), using relatively large samples of patients with schizophrenia (n=54) and bipolar illness (n=48), studied the volume and asymmetry of various brain structures that have been shown to be abnormal in previous imaging studies. They found that bipolar patients did not differ from the controls except for a somewhat smaller right hippocampus. Like normal controls, patients with schizophrenia and males with bipolar illness had right temporal lobes larger than the left. Bipolar female patients, on the other hand, did not display this asymmetry, a finding that the investigators suggest could be due to a neurodevelopmental abnormality mediated through environmental, genetic or hormonal influences. As Nasrallah (1991) points out, the structural brain abnormalities found in bipolar illness have generally not been seen as evidence for a neurodevelopmental abnormality, as they have in schizophrenia. Both neuroanatomy and neurodevelopment have been relatively neglected in research on bipolar illness, and the work that has been done is difficult to interpret. The advent of functional MRI technology should, in the near future, give us a clearer picture of possible brain abnormalities in manic-depressive illness and their possible neurodevelopmental implications.

At the cellular level, attempts to understand the mechanism of antidepressant and mood stabilizing agents are proceeding rapidly and may lead to a better understanding of the specific genetic vulnerability in recurrent affective illness. Of particular interest in recent years have been second-messenger systems, particularly mechanisms involving the G proteins, cyclic AMP cascade and phosphatidylinositol (PI). For example, Berridge and colleagues proposed that lithium restores normal neural activity by selectively suppressing PI in the most overactive receptor-mediated neuronal pathways (Berridge 1989; Berridge et al. 1989). Down regulation of this second-messenger system could correct an imbalance, dampening an overly excited system, stimulating an inhibited one, and exerting no effect on a normally balanced system. Key to this is the fact that lithium's effect is proportional to the level of activation of the PI system.

Most recently, research has focused on the effects of mood-altering agents on gene expression. For example lithium can activate the immediate early gene transcription factor, c-*fos* by protein kinase C (PKC), an enzyme found throughout the body with rich concentrations in the brain. For various studies have shown that lithium selectively activates the PKC signal transduction pathway – an important distinction, since *fos* appears to serve as a "master switch" inducing many different secondary changes in cellular function.

Natural course is the key to understanding the recurrence of manic-depressive illness, and two of the most interesting hypotheses about the illness have used longitudinal clinical observations as a starting point. One hypothesis posits that the episodic nature of most affective illness, perhaps the cycles of the bipolar subtypes, reflects a disturbance in the regulation of biological rhythms, especially circadian (24-h) rhythms. The second theorizes that the inherent cyclicity of mood disorders may involve a process roughly analogous to electrical kindling, whereas mania more closely resembles the related process of behavioral sensitization to psychostimulants (e.g., cocaine).

It is now well established that the endogenous pacemaker in mammals is located in the suprachiasmatic nuclei (SCN) of the hypothalamus, temporally ordering a wide range of central nervous system (CNS) functions. My colleagues and I have speculated elsewhere (Wehr and Goodwin 1983; Goodwin and Jamison 1990) that the biological clock's overriding organizing function may be dysregulated in manic-depressive illness. A primary circadian disturbance could produce widespread dysregulation within and between the many physiological systems known to show circadian, infradian (more than a day), and ultradian (less than a day) rhythmicity. They include neurotransmitter systems (e.g., Healy 1987), the hypothalamic-pituitary-adrenal axis and other aspects of neuroendocrine function (e.g., Angeli et al. 1992), the immune system (e.g., Maes et al. 1991), and other biological processes symptomatic of manic-depressive illness, such as sleep patterns and food intake.

Periodic oscillations are ubiquitous throughout the plant and animal world and at all levels of biological organization. More than one oscillator appears to regulate rhythmic processes and can become desynchronized, even, as was recently demonstrated, within a single-cell organism (Roenneberg and Morse 1993). Consistent with this finding, Wehr et al. (1993), in experiments with normal human subjects, found evidence that the circadian system is regulated by multiple oscillators. This conclusion was inferred from the fact that, as the seasons and the photoperiod changed, various rhythms (temperature, thyrotropin, melatonin) shifted as well, but not in synchrony. Sleep time also changed with the photoperiod. Based on these findings, Wehr and his colleagues hypothesize that sleep-cycle abnormalities are involved in the pathogenesis of bipolar manic-depressive illness. As patients switch from mania to depression or vice versa, their nocturnal sleep time grows longer and shorter. Changes in mood accompany those sleep changes – just as sleep deprivation can quickly lift the mood of a depressed patient. Understanding the mechanism of those changes could clarify the pathological process in affective illness.

Recurrent affective illness itself constitutes an infradian rhythm, a cyclicity that could arise by way of the curious properties of rhythms. Computer simulations have suggested that coupling of "cells" that oscillate in an apparently chaotic pattern can generate increased periodicity in the resulting "tissue" (Klevecz and Bolen 1992).

Conversely, coupling periodic oscillators can lead to the expression of strange or chaotic behavior in the population of cells. These simulations, built on the results of basic research into period mutants in *Drosophila*, the common fruit fly, suggest that a chaotic ultradian oscillator may actually underlie the circadian clock. By analogy, circadian dysregulation (in a sense, a "chaotic" oscillator) could conceivably lead to the longer-term rhythmicity of manic-depressive illness. This type of regulatory model is in keeping with the suggestions made by Mandell (1985), who argues that to predict the dynamics of a complex system such as the brain requires more attention to the stability of the system and less to reductionistic linear constructs.

Earlier, Halberg (1968) suggested one possible pattern of circadian rhythm dysregulation: free-running rhythms that are not entrained to the 24-h day cycle, gradually going in and out of phase with other circadian rhythms that remain synchronized with the day/night cycle. This internal desynchronziation can create what has been called a beat phenomenon, analogous to the audible beat produced by two tuning forks of slightly different frequencies. Further elaborating on the free-running hypothesis, Wehr and Goodwin (1983) and Kripke (1983) suggested that stable depression might occur in patients in whom an overly fast, intrinsic pacemaker rhythm causes circadian rhythms to become abnormally but stably advanced relative to the day/night cycle. Cyclic depression, on the other hand, may result from an overly fast rhythm escaping from entrainment; it then free-runs, advancing repeatedly through 360° relative to the day/night cycle. The possibilty of such free-running circadian rhythms has far-reaching implications for research on manic-depressive illness. Not only could such a mechanism drive the dramatic cyclicity observed in some bipolar patients, but it could also result in epiphenomena that are misinterpreted as biological correlates of changes in the mood cycle.

Animal data indicate that the frequency of circadian oscillators and seasonal photoperiodic mechanisms are under genetic control. Whether genetic factors contribute to variability in the phase position of circadian rhythms among manic-depressive patients is unknown. Only a few clinical studies have attempted to trace possible genetic influences on cyclicity. Some data suggest that rapid-cycling bipolar disorder shares the same genetic substrate with nonrapid-cycling disorder. Winokur and Kadrmas (1989), on the other hand, found a strong relationship between many episodes in bipolar patients (three or more) and a history of bipolar illness and remitting affective disorder in first-degree relatives. They suggest that what is inherited may be an episodic course, not bipolar illness – a speculation that deserves further exploration.

Animal research offers intriguing clues to the effects of such rhythmic abnormalities. Among the most important developments to date is the serendipitous identification of an animal model of a genetically abnormal fast biological clock. Ralph and Menaker (1988) found that a single-gene mutation shortened the circadian period in a golden hamster, a mammal of considerable interest in chronobiology because of its unusually narrow free-running period of circadian rhythmicity. Through subsequent breeding, the investigators were able to characterize the mutant allele, *tau*, and found that animals who inherited it from both parents had free-running periods of 20 h. Unlike normal hamsters, the mutant animals were seldom able to become entrained to 24-h light cycles. In response to single light pulses, they made phase shifts in both directions – delays and advances – a finding that may suggest that the mutant gene weakens the coupling between oscillators comprising the circadian pacemaker (Menaker and Refinetti 1992). The mutant hamsters, which showed a few behavioral characteristics reminiscent of manic-depressive illness, represent the first mammalian model of genetic disturbance in biological rhythms, a development that could help to clarify the role of the circadian system in regulating normal CNS functioning. Preliminary evidence suggests a similar speeding up of the circadian clock in rapid-cycling bipolar patients under free-running conditions. Another hypthesis put forth to explain clinical findings posits that manic-deppressive patients, like hamsters with the *tau* mutation, have a decreased capacity for entrainment.

Seasonal rhythms in neurotransmitter and neuroendocrine function also influence the course of illness and response to medications. A large literature has now accumulated documenting seasonal variations in several biological systems, and a few studies have related these rhythms to clinical characteristics. In recent reports on human subjects, for example, seasonal variations were observed in the volume and vasopressin cell number of the SCN (Hofman et al. 1993) and in whole blood and platelet serotonin content (Mann et al. 1992).

The role of stress in the onset of affective episodes has been a focus of depression research for years. Two recent developments have again put stress research in the center of efforts to understand the pathophysiology of affective disorders. First, Kendler et al. (1993) have extensively studied a large cohort of female twins ($n = 1030$), 57% of whom are monozygotic. After factoring out genetic contributions using multiple regression and relative risk analyses, they found that the presence of recent stressful events was the single most powerful predictor of major depression.

The focus of research on stress in affective disorder has begun to shift to a greater emphasis on understanding the impact of recurrent stressors. Here the most extensive developed model is that of kindling/sensitization, developed most comprehensively by Post et al. (1981) National Institute of Mental Health (NIMH). Initially proposed as a way of understanding certain features of rapidly cycling bipolar disorder, the model may also have general relevance to recurrent pathologies, such as posttraumatic stress disorder. Classically, kindling refers to the process by which intermittent (but not chronic) subthreshold stimuli, either electrical or chemical, eventually produce neuronal depolarization responses of increasing intensity even though the size of the stimulus is held constant (Goddard et al. 1969). When the repeated stimuli are applied to the limbic system, eventually limbic seizures ensue and characteristically they continue indefinitely after the removal of the stimulus. Apparently, permanent changes has been introduced; it is as if the neuronal system has developed a molecular memory of the stimuli, and responds accordingly.

In Post's model, a kindling-like process is evoked to account for important features of the natural course of recurrent affective illness, in particular, the rapidly cycling bipolar disorder. Thus, while the onset of early episodes appears to be precipitated by immediate prior stressors, their importance diminishes with each subsequent episode, so that by the fourth or fifth episode there is, on average, no longer any evidence for stress precipitation (reviewed in Goodwin and Jamison 1990; Post 1992); that is, the course of the illness has become autonomous. Related to this are experimental observations in animals (reviewed by Post and Weiss 1995) suggesting that the "scars" left by earlier episodes are directly linked to the increasingly vulnerability to episodes and the decreasing importance of external stressors. The emerging appreciation of the fact that "episodes beget episodes" is translated into a new emphasis on early aggressive and continuous prophylaxis.

Furthermore, a kindling-like process could account for the fact that the severity of untreated recurrent affective episodes worsens over time, especially in bipolar patients (Goodwin and Jamison 1990). Third, kindling could explain the tendency for the interval between affective episodes (i.e., the cycle length) to shorten over time, as well as the progressively shorter latency between the onset of an episode and its peak severity (Goodwin and Jamison 1990). Finally, as suggested by Gold et al. (1988), a kindling-like process is consistent with findings that stressful experiences in childhood comprise part of the vulnerability to affective disorders in adulthood (Cummings and Davies 1994). A related model for long-term increases in neuronal responsivity to stimuli is the process of sensitization to recurrently administered psychomotor stimulants such as cocaine (Post et al. 1981). Apparently medicated by different mechanisms, the overall effect of sensitization is both similar to and distinct from that of kindling (Post and Weiss 1995).

One of the most interesting features of the kindling process in animals is age dependency – young animals are more sensitive than adult animals; that is, compared to adults, kindling can be introduced in young animals with stimuli of considerably less intensity (Fanelli and McNamara 1986). Typically the age of onset of bipolar disorder is the teens or early twenties – which is the period of greatest vulnerability to stimulus (stress)-induced kindling (at least in experimental animals). The implications of this for early detection and aggressive treatment can hardly be overstated (Post 1992). It is especially important to emphasize this because the field of child and adolescent psychiatry has traditionally been somewhat resistant to diagnosis ("labeling") to treat with medication. Furthermore, if a kindling-like process is involved in the initiation of the illness, then it is possible that the illness might be prevented by preventing the age-dependent kindling process from developing in vulnerable individuals. The administration of acute kindling agents (i.e., carbamazepine) prior to the onset of symptoms is a possible prevention technique. By extension of the animal data, one of us (Goodwin 1993) has hypothesized that once a genetically vulnerable person passes through the age of risk for onset of the illness (age-dependent kindling), the likelihood of the illness appearing is sufficiently low that lifelong maintenance medication is less likely to be necessary. Given ethical concerns about the administration of drugs in the absence of chemical disorder, the evolution of this hypothesis will probably have to await development of markers that could, with reasonable sensitivity and specificity, identify those children very likely to develop the illness once they reach the age of risk.

New evidence from neuroscience has underlined the importance of taking a long view of affective and other mental illnesses. Because the environment can alter gene expression even before birth, renewed emphasis on developmental processes is essential. So are longitudinal studies in all domains of clinical research. We simply cannot continue to sample some biological variable only while patients are in the midst of an episode of illness. If genetic studies can help to identify individuals who are at maximum risk of developing the illness, prospective longitudinal studies can help to clarify the interaction of environmental/experiential factors. In the meantime, greater attention to individual differences and less dependence on group means could help us to understand more about how stressful experience energizes some and causes illness in othes.[1]

Obviously, knowledge from such studies has important public health implications. I have never been more optimistic about the potential of science to aid our patients. Already we can predict that early and continuing treatment can minimize the ravages of the illness. Fuller understanding of the long-term pathophysiological process should make it possible to design treatment strategies that allow vulnerable individuals to live – free of the pain and scars of this serious mental illness.

References

Altshuler LL (1993) Bipolar disorder: are repeated episodes associated with neuroanatomic and cognitive changes? Biol Psychiatry 33: 563–565

Andreasen NC, Swayze V II, Flaum M, Alliger R, Cohen G (1990) Ventricular abnormalities in affective disorder: clinical and demographic correlates. Am J Psychiatry 147: 893–900

Angeli A, Gatti G, Masera R (1992) Chronobiology of hypothalamic-pituitary-adrenal and renin-angiotensin-aldosterone systems. In: Touitou Y, Haus E (eds) Biological rhythms in clinical and laboratory medicine. Springer, Berlin Heidelberg New York, pp 292–314

Arana GW, Pearlman C, Shader RI (1985) Alprazolam-induced mania: two clinical cases. Am J Psychiatry 142: 368–369

Berridge MJ (1989) The Albert Lasker Medical Awards. Inositol triphosphate, calcium, lithium, and cell signaling. JAMA 262: 1834–1841

Berridge MJ, Downes CP, Hanley MR (1989) Neural and developmental actions of lithium: a unifying hypothesis. Cell 59: 411–419

Breier A, Albus M, Pickar D, Zahn TP, Wolkowitz OM, Paul SM (1987) Controllable and uncontrollable stress in humans: alterations in mood and neuroendocrine and psychophysiological function. Am J Psychiatry 144: 1419–1425

Chaouloff F (1993) Physiopharmacological interactions between stress hormones and central serotonergic systems. Brain Res Rev 18: 1–32

Cummings EM, Davies PT (1994) Maternal depression and child development. J Child Psychol Psychiatry 35 (1): 73–113

Divish MM, Sheftel G, Boyle A, Kalasapudi VD, Papolos DF, Lachman HM (1991) Differential effect of lithium on fos protooncogene expression mediated by receptor and postreceptor activators of protein kinase C and cyclic adenosine monophosphate: model for its antimanic action. J Neurosci Res 28: 40–48

Dupont RM, Jernigan TL, Gillin JC, Butters N, Delis DC, Hesselink JR (1987) Subcortical signal hyperintensities in bipolar patients detected by MRI. Psychiatry Res 21: 357–358

Fanelli RJ, McNamara JO (1986) Effects of age on kindling and kindled seizure-induced increase of benzodiazepine receptor binding. Brain Res 362 (1): 17–22

Goddard GV, McIntyre DC, Leech CK (1969) A permanent change in brain function resulting from daily electrical stimulation. Exp Neurol 25: 295–330

Gold PW, Goodwin FK, Chrousos GP (1988) Clinical and biochemical manifestations of stress: relation to the neurobiology of stress. Part II. N Engl J Med 319: 413–420

Goodwin FK, Jamison KR (1990) Manic-depressive illness. Oxford University Press, New York

Goodwin FK (1993) Integrated perspectives on the treatment of depression. Foundation for Advanced Education in the Sciences Psychopharmacology in Practice: Clinical and Research Update, Bethesda

Gurguis GNM, Meador-Woodruff JH, Haskett RF, Greden JF (1990) Multiplicity of depressive episodes: phenomenological and neuroendocrine correlates. Biol Psychiatry 27: 1156–1164

Halberg G (1968) Physiologic considerations underlying thythmometry, with special reference to emotional illness. In: DeAjuriaguerra J (ed) Cycles biologiques et psychiatrie. Masson, Paris pp 73–126. Symposium Bel-Air III, Geneva

1 See Salmon and Stanford (1992) and accompanying commentaries for an interesting discussion of this point.

Healy D (1987) Rhythm and blues: neurochemical, neuropharmacological and neuropsychological implications of a hypothesis of circadian rhythm dysfunction in the affective disorders. Psychopharmacology (Berl) 93: 271–285
Hofman MA, Purba JS, Swaab DF (1993) Annual variations in the vasopressin neuron population of the human suprachiasmatic nucleus. Neuroscience 53: 1103–1112
Kendler KS, Kessler RC, Neale MC et al. (1993) The prediction of major depression in women. Am J Psychiatry 150: 1139–1148
Klevecz RR, Bolen JL Jr (1992) Dynamic analysis of period mutants in Drosophila: how a precise circadian clock might emerger from a tissue composed of chaotic cellular oscillators. In: Young MW (ed) Molecular genetics of biological rhythms. Dekker, New York, pp 221–253
Kripke DF (1983) Phase-advance theories for affective illnesses. In: Wehr TA, Goodwin FK (eds) Circadian rhythms in psychiatry. Boxwood, Pacific Grove, pp 41–69
McEwen BS, Angulo J, Cameron H, Chao HM, Daniels D, Gannon MN, Gould E, Mendelson S, Sakai R, Spencer R, Woolley C (1992) Paradoxical effects of adrenal steroids on the brain: Protection versus degeneration. Biol Psychiatry 31: 177–199
Maes M, Bosman E, Suy E, Minner B, Raus G (1991) A further exploration of the relationship between immune parameters and the HPA axis in depressed patients. Psychol Med 21: 313–320
Mandell AJ (1985) From molecular biological simplification to more realistic central nervous system dynamics: an overview. In: Michels R, Cavenar JO Jr, Brodie HKH, Cooper AM, Guze SB, Judd LL, Klerman GL, Solnit AJ (eds) Psychiatry, vol 3. Lippincott, London
Manji HK, Lenox RH (1995) Long term action of lithium: a role for transcriptional and posttranscriptional factors regulated by protein kinase. C. Synapse (in press)
Mann JJ, McBride PA, Anderson GM, Mieczkowski TA (1992) Platelet and whole blood serotonin content in depressed inpatients: correlations with acute and life-time psychopathology. Biol Psychiatry 32: 243–257
Menaker M, Refinetti R (1992) The tau mutation in golden hamsters. In: Young MW (ed) Molecular genetics of biological rhythms. Dekker, New York, pp 255–269
Nasrallah HA (1991) Neurodevelopment aspects of bipolar affective disorder. Biol Psychiatry 29: 1–2
Post RM (1992) Transduction of psychosocial stress into the neurobiology of recurrent affective disorder. Am J Psychiatry 149: 999–1010
Post RM, Weiss SRB (1992) Endogenous biochemical abnormalities in affective illness: therapeutic versus pathogenic. Biol Psychiatry 32: 469–484
Post RM, Weiss SRB (1995) The neurobiology of treatment-resistant mood disorders. In: Bloom FE, Kupfer DJ (eds) Psychopharmacology: the fourth generation of progress. Raven, New York
Post RM, Lockfeld A, Squillace KM, Contel NR (1981) Drug-environment interaction: context dependency of cocaine-induced behavioral sensitization. Life Sci 28: 755–760
Ralph MR, Menaker M (1988) A mutation of the circadian system in golden hamsters. Science 241: 1225–1227
Roenneberg T, Morse D (1993) Two circadian oscillators in one cell. Nature 362: 362–364
Salmon P, Stanford SC (1992) Critique: research strategies for decoding the neurochemical basis of resistance to stress. J Psychopharmacol 6: 1–7
Strakowski SM, Wilson DR, Tohen M, Woods BT, Douglass AW, Stoll AL (1993) Structural brain abnormalities in first-episode mania. Biol Psychiatry 33: 602–609
Swayze VW, Andreasen NC, Alliger RJ, Ehrhardt JC, Yuh WTC (1992a) Structural brain abnormalities in bipolar affective disorder: ventricular enlargement and focal signal hyperintensities. Arch Gen Psychiatry 47: 1054–1059
Swayze VW, Andreasen NC, Alliger RJ, Yuh WTC, Ehrhardt JC (1992b) subcortical and temporal structures in affective disorder and schizophrenia: a magnetic resonance imaging study.
Wehr TA, Goodwin FK (1983) Biological rhythms in manic-depressive illness. In: Wehr TA, Goodwin FK (eds) Circadian rhythms in psychiatry. Boxwood, Pacific Grove
Wehr TA, Moul DE, Barbato G, Giesen HA, Seidel JA, Barker C, Bender C (1993) Conservation of photoperiod-responsive mechanisms in human beings. Am J Physiol 34: 846–857
Welsh DK, Moore-Ede MC (1990) Lithium lengthens circadian period in a diurnal primate Saimiri sciureus. Biol Psychiatry 28: 117–126
Winokur G, Kadrmas A (1989) A polyepisodic course in bipolar illness: possible clinical relationship. Compr Psychiatry 30: 121–127
Woods BT, Yurgelun-Todd, Benes FM, Frankenburg FR, Pope HG Jr., McSparren J (1990) Progressive ventricular enlargement in schizophrenia: comparison to bipolar affective disorder and correlation with clinical course. Biol Psychiatry 27: 341–352

New Findings in the Genetics of Bipolar Illness*

E.S. GERSHON

Introduction

Traditionally, the genetics of psychiatric disorders consisted of the results of twin, adoption, and family studies. The outcome of such studies in bipolar illness consists of evidence that a genetic component of liability is operating, as well as definitions of the inherited phenotype, and morbid risk estimates. What has *not* come out of these studies is subdivson of the observed illness into distinct genetic subclasses, or an inherited pathophysiology. Recent progress in genetic linkage studies of this disorder, however, leads one to expect that susceptibility mutations and molecular diagnostic subclasses will soon be discovered.

Bipolar illness, as we now think of it, falls into the genetic classification of common diseases with complex inheritance, meaning that a single gene cannot account for all the cases of a disease, even within a single family. As in other members of this class of diseases, progress toward identifying specific susceptibility genes has become possible with the advances in DNA technology, and in analytic methodologies which are robust to this type of inheritance. Of particular importance is the emergence of a very dense and highly informative linkage map. To take advantage of these technological advances, a thorough knowledge is needed of the diagnostic epidemiology of the illness, and families must be identified and studied who can efficiently generate information on linkage or association of particular genes with illness.

Genetic Diagnostic Epidemiology of Bipolar (BP) Illness

Coaggregation of BP and Related Diagnoses in Families

The twin, family, and adoption studies of BP have been extensively reviewed elsewhere (Nurnberger et al. 1994; Gershon and Nurnberger 1995) and these have led to a general consensus that there is a familial aggregation of major depression (unipolar mood disorder; UP) and schizoaffective (SA) disorder in families of BP patients, as compared with control rates.

Relatives of BP patients have more BP illness, but about the same UP illness, as relatives of UP patients. This is one of the findings that have led to the conclusion that

* This manuscript includes updated materials from Gershon ES (in press) Recent developments in genetics of bipolar illness. In: Gessa GL, Fratta L, Serra G (eds) *Depression: neurobiology, pharmacology and clinic: Proceedings of the 8th Sardinian Conference on Neuroscience*, Raven, New York.

there is an overlap of inherited susceptibility to BP and UP illness, although of course one is not assuming that there is only one inherited susceptibility to either disorder.

SA disorder, it is generally agreed, is associated with BP illness in many families. The identical twins of SA patients tend to have the same disorder but the first-degree relatives have a considerable frequency of affective disorder, both UP and BP, and also small but consistent increases in SA disorder an schizophrenia, as compared with controls (Table 1). The problem is that SA disorder is also found in relatives of schizophrenics; the family data are reviewed elsewhere (Nurnberger et al. 1994; Cloninger 1994; Crow 1994). The picture is further complicated by recent studies in which major depression is increased in relatives of schizophrenia (Maier et al. 1993; Nurnberger et al. 1994).

Table 1. Lifetime prevalence of psychotic and affective disorders in first-degree relatives of patients and controls

Proband diagnosis	No. of relatives	Schizo-phrenia	SA (chronic)	SA (acute)	Other psychosis	Bipolar (I and II)	Unipolar
Schizophrenia	108	3.1	0	5.0	3.1	1.3	14.7
Schizoaffective (chronic psychosis)	129	1.7	2.5	0	6.7	8.8	9.3
Schizoaffective (acute psychosis)	69	4.9	1.6	5.8	3.2	11.7	16.4
Bipolar	738	0.3	0.1	1.6	0.6	7.2	14.9
Unipolar	165	0	0	0.7	4.4	2.9	16.7
Controls	380	0.6	0	0.6	1.2	0.3	6.7

Prevalences are morbid risk (percent). SA, schizoaffective disorder. (Data from Gershon et al., 1982, 1988)

There are differences of opinion over whether these and other data constitute evidence for genetic overlap of BP and schizophrenia, or whether the Kraepelinian dichotomy is valid and these overlapping diagnoses have indeterminate origin (Cloninger 1994; Crow 1994). As a practical matter for genetic linkage and association studies, the investigator must balance the added statistical power of including schizoaffectives and unipolars as affected in BP families, against the risk that one is including, as affected, persons with a different genetic basis for their disease. It appears to us acceptable, in families with more than one BP person, to consider BP illness to be a core entity, with UP illness and SA disorder being the outcome when additional nonshared genetic or environmental features are present.

Cohort Effect

People born in the decades starting approximately 1940 have a higher lifetime prevalence of affective disorders than people born earlier, as reviewed elsewhere (Nurnberger et al. 1994). In our own data on relatives of BP and SA patients, the age at onset for BP and SA disorders has become earlier and the total lifetime prevalence appears likely to be much higher in the cohorts born since 1940 (Gershon et al. 1987).

In our original description of this finding, we interpreted it as a gene-environmental interaction, since the increased rates were far higher in relatives of patients than in population data, and it did not appear that genetic change could occur so rapidly (from one generation to the next).

Recently, a new form of genetic change which occurs rapidly within predisposed families has been described. Expansion of DNA trinucleotide repeat sequences can occur as germ cells are formed and in early stages of embryonic development. This has been found to be the disease mutation in several CNS-related diseases, including Huntington's disease and fragile X syndrome mental retardation. A clinical feature of these diseases is *anticipation*, which refers to an increase in disease severity and/or earlier age of onset in successive generations. It has recently been argued (McInnis et al. 1993) that anticipation occurs in BP illness, and that trinucleotide repeat expansion may thus prove to be the basis of the genetic predisposition. The argument on anticipation is not compelling, since in family data it would appear to be impossible *not* to confound anticipation with a birth-cohort effect from another cause.

Other interpretations have also been offered. It has been argued that the entire finding is an artifact of recollection (Simon and von Korff 1992); this argument would not be valid for studies of contemporaneously collected data on BP illness, such as that of Angst (1985).

Detection of Susceptibility Genes Through Linkage

Segregation Analysis

The inheritance patterns of BP in families do not fit simple Mendelian transmission (they do not segregate in families as simple recessives or dominants). Complex segregation analyses (that is, analyses with variable penetrance, presence of multifactorial inheritance, etc.) have not, so far, yielded a uniquely supported set of genetic transmission parameters (penetrance and allele frequencies), in the sense that there is significant rejection of all but one set of parameter values in a particular set of nested genetic models, as reviewed elsewhere (Nurnberger et al. 1994). More recent analyses give similar outcomes. Curtis et al. (1993b) recently did segregation analysis on five selected Icelandic pedigrees. It is not clear whether the pedigrees were selected *because* they appeared to have dominant transmission. Dominant inheritance gave an equally likely fit to the mixed model, when bipolar [only] was considered affected. The mixed model fit better when unipolar illness was included as affected.

Risch (1990) has demonstrated that some conclusions on inheritance can be drawn, even though segregation analyses are not conclusive about an illness. When a single gene or multilocus additive genes cause illness susceptibility, the risk ratio (risk to relatives vs population risk; lambda) progressively decreases, according to a fixed ratio, as one examines more distantly related relatives. For example, the observed value of the expression lambda-1 should be twice as high in monozygotic twins as in dizygotic twins. In schizophrenia, the risk to monozygotic twins is too much greater than that to siblings to fit these types of inheritance. Although Risch does not discuss BP illness, the same conclusions would apply. One would look for oligogenic inheritance with interactions between susceptibility loci. These may prove to be detectable through linkage analysis methods which do not require that genetic transmission parameters be specified, such as the affected-sib-pair method (ASP; Suarez et al. 1978), or the affected-pedigree-member method (APM; Weeks and Lange 1988).

Results of Genomic Scanning Linkage Studies in Bipolar Illness

The strategy of systematic genomic scanning for a susceptibility locus to bipolar illness has not yet been widely applied. The first comprehensive map using DNA marker loci was reported by Donnis-Keller et al. in 1987 Since then, the informativeness of DNA markers has greatly improved, particularly with the development of microsatellite markers; gaps have been filled; and the density of the map has increased. A recent map has 2066 microsatellite markers, with only modest gaps (Gyapay et al. 1994).

Understandably, the number of bipolar pedigrees studied with many markers is modest; no group of investigators has yet reported that it has completed its scan of the entire genome. Preliminary results of genomic scans have been reported by several investigators. In the Old Order Amish, following the failure of replication of the reported linkage on chromosome 11p (Kelsoe et al. 1989). Ginns et al. (1992) reported on 250 restriction fragment length polymorphism (RFLP) markers and Pakstis et al. (1991) reported on 185 markers, without linkage detection. Curtis et al. (1993b) reported on regions of chromosome 11p, 11q, 8q, 5q, 9q, and Xq in five Icelandic pedigrees, where linkage was not found. Coon et al. (1993) examined eight U.S. pedigrees at 328 marker loci. Again, linkage was not detected. A marker locus on the distal portion of 5q, a region containing several receptor genes, gave a slightly positive logarithm of differences (lod) score, but examination in that region of the D_1 receptor and a closely linked marker (CRI-L1200) gave very negative lod scores (Jensen et al. 1992).

Straub et al. (1994) reporting on 47 U.S. and Israeli pedigrees, have applied up to 157 marker loci per pedigree. One family had a lod score of 3.4 at locus PFKL on chromosome 21q, under dominant inheritance, although the multipoint lod score in that region was negative. Analysis by the parameter-free APM method showed statistically significant evidence for linkage in the pedigree series as a whole. This implies a susceptibility gene with small effect, possibly as part of an oligogenic inheritance system.

My colleagues and I have been studying a series of 22 U.S. pedigrees (Berrettini et al. 1991). Including a manuscript submitted for publication (Berrettini et al. submitted) 537 loci have been studied (Gejman et al. 1990, 1993; Detera-Wadleigh et al. 1992, 1994; Berrettini et al. 1990). The locus reported by Straub et al. (1994) is not linked to illness in our series (S. Detera-Wadleigh, unpublished data).

In one region on chromosome 18, Berrettini et al. (1994) observed lod scores >1 for several pedigrees in this series, with different pedigrees having these scores under dominant and under recessive inheritance. The highest lod score for one pedigree was 2.3 under recessive inheritance. Analysis was performed by parameter-free methods. ASP and multipoint APM showed statistically significant evidence for linkage (Table 2). To be established as a linkage, of course, replication is required.

Table 2. Affected-sib-pair analysis on chromosome 18

Marker locus	ILL: BP & SA (Model I)		ILL: BP, SA & UP (Model II)	
	% IBD	*p* value	% IBD	*p* value
S59	.54	.173	.51	.369
S170	.53	.28	.53	.163
S62	.53	.162	.57	.002
S21	.55	.066	.57	.0013
S37	.56	.029	.56	.0108
S32	.61	.0003	.62	<.00001
S453	.53	.162	.54	.063
S53	.58	.0175	.54	.041
S40	.57	.051	.58	.0046
S45	.58	.0089	.57	.002
S44	.53	.20	.55	.029
S66	.58	.044	.56	.028
S56	.60	.0043	.57	.0067
S47	.53	.163	.52	.159
S35	.50	1.0	.51	.296
S64	.55	.065	.51	.268
S31	.52	.288	.50	.478
S27	.51	.439	.49	1.0

P values adjusted for multiple sib-pairs within sibships by reducing the degrees of freedom in the *t*-test to the number of independent comparisons (*r*-1 for each sibship, where *r* is the number of affected sibs). % IBD, proportion of marker alleles identical by descent in affected sib pairs. (Data from Berrettini et al., submitted.)

O.C. Stine et al. (Stine and DePaulo 1994) recently reported a replication of the linkage, in an ASP analysis of an independently collected pedigree series, with results quite similar to those in Table 2. This strengthens the conclusion that the linkage is valid.

Replication is not necessarily to be expected in every data set, however. In pedigrees simulated under additive oligogenic inheritance with four to ten loci, where any combination greater than a threshold number of "susceptibility" alleles at these loci can lead to a trait, Suarez et al. (1994) have demonstrated that a much smaller sample is needed initially to detect linkage to one of the trait loci than to replicate linkage to that locus. This result is intuitively reasonable, since any of the four to ten loci can be the first to be detected, but in any replication sample of the same size, the chances that one *specific* locus will be detected is considerably smaller than the probability than any one of four to ten may be detected.

Linkage Studies of Candidate Genes

This strategy may appear more appealing than genomic scanning in common diseases until one asks, in BP illness, on what basis is any gene a candidate. As reviewed elsewhere (Nurnberger et al. 1994), the pathophysiology of illness is not well enough elucidated to give promising candidate genes. However, based on the neuropharmacology of treatment agents for depression and for psychosis, dopamine and serotonin receptor genes and transporter genes have been appealing to many psychiatric geneticists.

Other candidate genes have been based on reported linkage findings and segregation analyses. It must be noted that some candidates have taken on a life of their own, even when the initial findings that generated the candidates have lapsed. This is true for the tip of the short arm of chromosome 11 (11p15). The genes in that small region include structural genes for insulin, tyrosine hydroxylase, the dopamine D_4 structural gene (DRD_4, and HRAS-1. It is generally agreed that linkage to BP illness in that region is not detectable, following the failure of replication of the linkage finding within the Old Order Amish pedigree where it was originally reported (Kelsoe et al. 1989), and the lack of other confirmatory reports. Linkage studies of the DRD_4 and of the enzyme tyrosine hydroxylase (or of the region spanning them) have continued to be reported (Sidenberg et al. 1994; Ewald et al. 1994; Kelsoe et al. 1993; De Bruyn et al. 1994; Curtis et al. 1993b; Mitchell et al. 1991; Byerley et al. 1992; Law et al. 1992; Pauls et al. 1991; Nanko et al. 1991; Mendlewicz et al. 1991); none have detected linkage.

Other dopamine receptor genes have been studied in bipolar illness, with linkage not detected to DRD_1 (Jensen et al. 1992; Coon et al. 1993; Mitchell et al. 1992; Nothen et al. 1992), DRD_2 (Ewald et al. 1994; Mitchell et al. 1992; Nothen et al. 1992; De Bruyn et al. 1994; Kelsoe et al. 1993; Curtis et al. 1993b), or DRD_3 (Mitchell et al. 1993; Rietschel et al. 1993; Shaikh et al. 1993).

Multiple candidates have been tested in large-scale genomic mapping scans of BP illness. Curtis et al. (1993b, a) report exclusion of linkage to genes for 5-HT_{1A} receptor, proenkephalin, and dopamine beta-hydroxylase. In my colleagues' and my own genomic scans and specific linkage studies of putative candidate genes, we have observed no linkage to these receptors: cannabinoid, 2-adrenergic (two separate genes), 1-adrenergic, 1- and 2-adrenergic, DRD_2 and human glucocorticoid receptor (reviewed in Gershon et al. 1994).

By and large, these exclusions of candidate genes are based on lod score computations, based on "reasonable" single locus models of BP illness. The validity of the exclusion depends on the model used. Since non-model-based analytic methods may be required for detection of linkage in very complex inheritance disorders, one must consider all these exclusions to be tentative.

X-Linkage

Linkage of BP illness to the color blindness genes (which are in tandem on the X chromosome (Xq28) was reported by Reich et al. in two families in 1969 and corroborated by multiple pedigree reports of Mendlewicz and Fleiss 1974 (Mendlewicz et al. 1972) and Baron et. al (1987) However, controversy arose. The original investigators were never able to find a pedigree which replicated the findings, the work of Mendlewicz and Fleiss had mapping inconsistencies (reviewed in (Gershon et al. 1994), and the report of Baron et al. (1987) was not replicated in follow-up of the same pedigrees (Baron et al. 1993; Gershon and Goldin 1994a). Other reports on this region were negative (see review in Gershon et al. (1994). Bocchetta et al. (1994) recently reported association of a G6PD allele with bipolar illness in Sardinia, but this has also been disputed (Gershon and Goldin 1994b; Baron et al. 1994).

In a more proximal region of the X chromosome (Xq27), centering on the locus for blood clotting factor IX (FIX), there have been several independent reports of linkage (Mendlewicz et al. 1987; Geller et al. 1994; Pekkarinen et al. 1994), and interesting reports of disease association/linkage in two families with a FIX disease (Christmas disease) (Gill et al. 1992; Craddock and Owen 1992) and one with fragile X syndrome (Jeffries et al. 1993). Other reports have been negative (Gejman et al. 1990).

With the recent positive reports, linkage to FIX appears to be a more supported hypothesis than the earlier data on Xq28. It should be noted that the FIX locus is far enough from the color blindness locus so that a disease in tight linkage with one would be unlinked to the other.

Association

Association exists when there is an allele which is more frequent in a series of unrelated patients as compared with population frequencies. Association may occur as follows: over the course of many generations, numerous recombinations occur on mutation-bearing chromosomes. These recombinations occur randomly along the chromosome, so even over many generations they are unlikely to occur within a specifiable very small region, such as the DNA sequences within 200 kb of an illness mutation. This region with no recombination over many generations is a region of linkage disequilibrium; if it contains polymorphic restriction enzyme recognition sites, an RFLP will be associated with the illness.

The chromosomal region scanned by an association test is usually much smaller than the region scanned by testing for linkage in pedigrees. Within a pedigree, which extends over only a few generations, there is a relatively large region around a disease mutation in which recombination does not occur during these few generations, or occurs infrequently. Thus, a marker at some distance will be coinherited (linked) with an illness gene in a family, but may not be associated with it in a large population.

Association is often a more powerful strategy statistically than linkage (Schaid and Sommer 1993; Gershon et al. 1989). This is generally true for association with a true disease mutation, even when the gene is playing only a modest role in illness susceptibility. For polymorphisms within a linkage region, association due to linkage disequilibrium may be detectable or not, depending on the number of ancestral disease mutations and other factors.

Some allelic associations have been reported with tyrosine hydroxylase, possibly stimulated initially by the report of linkage to an adjacent marker (insulin) on chromosome 11p15, which is discussed above. Following an initial positive association report (Leboyer et al. 1990) of bipolar illness with tyrosine hydroxylase, a series of negative studies was reported (Gill et al. 1991), and there has been an additional recent negative report (Inayama et al. 1993).

Associations have also been sought at the end of the long arm of the X chromosome, as well, again because of linkage reports. The gene responsible for the fragile X syndrome, FMR1, which has been hypothesized to lead also to affective disorder, has been studied but no abnormality was detected in bipolar illness (Craddock et al. 1994).

Discussion

With the improvements in the informativeness and density of the genetic linkage map, and the important increases in the number of pedigrees being collected and the number of laboratories doing molecular studies in this illness, one can be optimistic about progress in the genetics of bipolar illness. Discovery of reproducible linkages to susceptibility genes appears to be assured, providing the susceptibility genes exist and enough "brute force" is applied. At this time, promising new linkage findings have been reported on chromosomes 18 and 21, which are awaiting replication studies. Several independent reports of linkage to FIX on the X chromosome are also promising.

Once linkage is demonstrated, the next goal is to identify the susceptibllity gene and its mutations within the linkage region. A general methodology for doing this in common disease with complex inheritance has not yet been developed. The problem is that one cannot use individual recombinants (persons who do not fit the linkage) even if they have illness, to rule out chromosomal regions from containing the susceptibility gene, when there is a substantial probability of phenocopies. In the case of chromosome 18, in addition, the region within which linkage is detectable is large (tens of centimorgans), too large to attempt to clone every gene within that region.

Thus, successes in detecting linkage will lead to new challenges, which may be equally difficult to overcome. Nonetheless, I expect that within the next decade there will be mutations identified in susceptibility genes, and that this will in turn lead to advances in diagnosis and treatment of this devastating disorder.

References

Angst J (1985) Switch from depression to mania: a record study over decades between 1920 and 1982. Psychopathology 18: 140–154

Baron M, Risch N, Hamberger R, Mandel B, Kushner S, Newman M, Drumer D, Belmaker RH (1987) Genetic linkage between X-chromosome markers and bipolar affective illness. Nature 326: 289–292

Baron M, Freimer NF, Risch N, Lerer B, Alexander JR, Straub RE, Asokan S, Das K, Peterson A, Amos J (1993) Diminished support for linkage between manic depressive illness and X-chromosome markers in three Israeli pedigrees [see comments]. Nature Genet 3: 49–55

Baron M, Straub RE, Lehner T, Endicott J, Ott J, Gilliam TC (1994) Correspondence: bipolar disorder and linkage to Xq28. Nature Genet 7: 461

Berrettini WH, Goldin LR, Gelernter J, Gejman PV, Gershon ES, Detera-Wadleigh SE (1990) X-chromosome markers and manic-depressive illness: rejection of linkage of Xq28 in nine bipolar pedigrees. Arch Gen Psychiatry 47: 366–373

Berrettini WH, Goldin LR, Martinez MM, Maxwell ME, Smith AL, Guroff JJ, Kazuba DM, Nurnberger JI Jr, Hamovit J, Simmons-Alling S, Muniec D, Choi H, York C, Robb AS, Gershon ES (1991) A bipolar pedigree series for genomic mapping of disease genes: diagnostic and analytic considerations. Psychiatr Genet 2: 125–160

Berrettini WH, Ferraro TN, Goldin LR, Weeks DE, Detera-Wadleigh S, Nurnberger JJ Jr, Gershon ES (1994) Chromosome 18 DNA markern and manic-depressive illness: evidence for a susceptibility gene. Proc Natl Acad Sci USA 91: 5918–5921

Bocchetta A, Piccardi MP, Del Zompo M (1994) Is bipolar disorder linked to Xq28? (Letter, comment). Nature Genet 6: 224

Byerley W, Plaetke R, Hoff M, Jensen S, Holik J, Reimherr F, Mellon C, Wender P, O'Connell P,

Leppert M (1992) Tyrosine hydroxylase gene not linked to manic-depression in seven of eight pedigrees. Hum Hered 42: 259–263
Cloninger CR (1994) Tests of alternative models of the relationship of schizophrenic and affective psychoses. In: Gershon ES, Cloninger CR (eds) Genetic approaches to mental disorders. American Psychiatric Press, Washington, pp 149–162 (American Psychopathological Association Series)
Coon H, Jensen S, Hoff M, Holik J, Plaetke R, Reimherr F, Wender P, Leppert M, Byerley W (1993) A genome-wide search for genes predisposing to manic-depression, assuming autosomal dominant inheritance. Am J Hum Genet 52: 1234–1249
Craddock N, Owen M (1992) Christmas disease and major affective disorder (Letter, comment). Br J Psychiatry 160: 715
Craddock N, Daniels J, McGuffin P, Owen M (1994) Variation at the fragile X locus does not influence susceptibility to bipolar disorder. Am J Med Genet 54: 141–143
Crow TJ (1994) The demise of the Kraepelinian binary system as a prelude to genetic advance. In: Gershon ES, Cloninger CR (eds) Genetic approaches to mental disorders. American Psychiatric, Washington, pp 163–202
Curtis D, Brynjolfsson J, Petursson H, Holmes DS, Sherrington R, Brett P, Rifkin L, Murphy P, Moloney E, Holmes SH (1993a) Segregation and linkage analysis in five manic depression pedigrees excludes the 5HT1a receptor gene (HTR1A). Ann Hum Genet 57: 27–39 [published erratum appears in Ann Hum Genet (1993) 57 (Pt 4): 311]
Curtis D, Sherrington R, Brett P, Holmes DS, Kalsi G, Brynjolfsson J, Petursson H, Rifkin L, Murphy P, Moloney E (1993b) Genetic linkage analysis of manic depression in Iceland. J R Soc Med 86: 506–510
De Bruyn A, Mendelbaum K, Sandkuijl LA, Delvenne V, Hirsch D, Staner L, Mendlewicz J, Van Broeckhoven C (1994) Nonlinkage of bipolar illness to tyrosine hydroxylase, tyrosinase, and D_2 and D_4 dopamine receptor genes on chromosome 11. Am J Psychiatry 151: 102–106
Detera-Wadleigh SD, Berrettini WH, Goldin LR, Martinez M, Hsieh WT, Hoehe MR, Encio IJ, Coffman D, Rollins DY, Muniec D (1992) A systematic search for a bipolar predisposing locus on chromosome 5. Neuropsychopharmacology 6: 219–229
Detera-Wadleigh SD, Hiseh WT, Berrettini WH, Goldin LR, Rollins DY, Muniec D, Grewal R, Guroff JJ, Turner G, Coffman D, Barrick J, Mills K, Murray J, Donohue SJ, Klein DC, Sanders J, Nurnberger JI Jr, Gershon ES (1994) Genetic linkage mapping for a susceptibility locus to bipolar illness: chromosomes 2,3,4,7,9,10p,11p,22, and Xpter. Am J Med Genet (Neuropsychiatr Genet 54: 206–218
Donis-Keller H, Green P, Helms C, Cartinour S, Weiffenbach B, Stephens K, Keith TP, Bowden DW, Smith DR, Lander ES, Botstein D, Akots G, Rediker KS, Gravius T (1987) A genetic linkage map of the human genome. Cell 51: 319–337
Ewald H, Mors O, Friedrich U, Flint T, Kruse T (1994) Exclusion of linkage between manic depressive illness and tyrosine hydroxylase and dopamine D_2 receptor genes. Psychiatr Genet 4: 13–22
Gejman PV, Detera-Wadleigh SD, Martinez MD, Berrettini WH, Goldin LR, Gelernter J, Hsieh WT, Gershon ES (1990) Manic depressive illness not linked to factor IX region in an independent series of pedigrees. Genomics 8: 648–655
Gejman PV, Martinez M, Cao Q, Friedman E, Berrettini WH, Goldin LR, Koroulakis P, Ames C, Lerman MA, Gershon ES (1993) Linkage analysis of fifty-seven microsatellite loci to bipolar disorder. Neuropsychopharmacology 9: 31–40
Geller B, Fox LW, Clark KA (1994) Rate and predictors of prepubenal bipolarity during follow-up of 6- to 12-year-old depressed children. J Am Acad Child Adolesc Psychiatry 33: 461–468
Gershon ES, Goldin LR (1994a) Replication of genetic linkage by follow-up of previously studied pedigrees. Am J Hum Genet 54: 715–718
Gershon ES, Goldin LR (1994b) Correspondence: bipolar disorder and linkage to Xq28. Nature Genet 7: 461–462
Gershon ES, Nurnberger JI Jr (1995) Bipolar illness. In: Oldham JM (ed) Review of psychiatry, vol 14. American Psychiatric Press, Washington
Gershon ES, Hamovit J, Guroff JJ, Dibble E, Leckman JF, Sceery W, Targum SD, Nurnberger JI Jr, Goldin LR, Bunney WE Jr (1982) A family study of schizoaffective, bipolar I, bipolar II, unipolar, and normal control probands. Arch Gen Psychiatry 39: 1157–1167
Gershon ES, Hamovit JR, Guroff JJ, Nurnberger JI Jr (1987) Birth-cohort changes in manic and depressive disorders in relatives of bipolar and schizoaffective patients. Arch Gen Psychiatry 44: 314–319
Gershon ES, DeLisi LE, Hamovit J, Nurnberger JI Jr, Maxwell ME, Schreiber J, Dauphinais D, Dingman CW, Guroff JJ (1988) A controlled family study of chronic psychoses: schizophrenia and schizoaffective disorder. Arch Gen Psychiatry 45: 328–336

Gershon ES, Martinez MM, Goldin LR, Gelernter J, Silver J (1989) Detection of marker associations with a dominant disease gene in genetically complex and heterogeneous diseases. Am J Hum Genet 45: 578–585

Gershon ES, Goldin LR, Martinez MM et al.(1994) Detecting discrete genes for susceptibility to bipolar disorder or schizophrenia. In: Gershon ES, Cloninger CR (eds) Genetic approaches to mental disorders. American Psychiatric Press, Washington, pp 205–230

Gill M, Castle D, Hunt N, Clements A, Sham P, Murray RM (1991) Tyrosine hydroxylase polymorphisms and bipolar affective disorder. J Psychiatr Res 25: 179–184

Gill M, Castle D, Duggan C (1992) Cosegregation of Christmas disease and major affective disorder in a pedigree (see comments). Br J Psychiatry 160: 112–114

Ginns El, Egeland JA, Allen CR, Pauls DL, Falls K, Keith TP, Paul SM (1992) Update on the search for DNA markers linked to manic-depressive illness in the Old Order Amish. J Psychiatr Res 26: 305–308

Gyapay G, Morissette J, Vignal A, Dib C, Fiznames C, Millasseau P, Marc S, Bernardi G, Lathrop M, Weissenbach J (1994) The 1993-94 Genethon human genetic linkage map. Nature Genet 7: 246–339

Inayama Y, Yoneda H, Sakai T, Ishida T, Kobayashi S, Nonomura Y, Kono Y, Koh J, Asaba H (1993) Lack of association between bipolar affective disorder and tyrosine hydroxylase DNA marker. Am J Med Genet 48: 87–89

Jeffries FM, Reiss AL, Brown WT, Meyers DA, Glicksman AC, Bandyopadhyay S (1993) Bipolar spectrum disorder and fragile X syndrome: a family study. Biol Psychiatry 33: 213–216

Jensen S, Plaetke R, Holik J, Hoff M, O'Connell P, Reimherr F, Wender P, Zhou QY, Civelli O, Litt M (1992) Linkage analysis of the D_1 dopamine receptor gene and manic depression in six families. Hum Hered 42: 269–275

Kelsoe JR, Ginns EI, Egeland JA, Gerhard DS, Goldstein AM, Bale SJ, Pauls DL, Long RT, Kidd KK, Conte G, Housman D, Housman DE, Paul SM (1989) Re-evaluation of the linkage relationship between chromosome 11p loci and the gene for bipolar affective disorder in the Old Order Amish. Nature 342: 238–243

Kelsoe JR, Kristbjanarson H, Bergesch P, Shilling P, Hirsch S, Mirow A, Moises HW, Helgason T, Gillin JC, Egeland JA (1993) A genetic linkage study of bipolar disorder and 13 markers on chromosome 11 including the D_2 dopamine receptor. Neuropsychopharmacology 9: 293–301

Law A, Richard CW, Cottingham RW Jr, Lathrop GM, Cox DR, Myers RM (1992) Genetic linkage analysis of bipolar affective disorder in an Old Order Amish pedigree. Hum Genet 88: 562–568

Leboyer M, Malafosse A, Boularand S et al. (1990) Tyrosine hydroxylase polymorphisms associated with manic-depressive illness. Lancet 335: 1219

Maier W, Lichtermann D, Minges J, Hallmayer J, Heun R, Benkert O, Levinson DF (1993) Continuity and discontinuity of affective disorders and schizophrenia. Results of a controlled family study. Arch Gen Psychiatry 50: 871–883

McInnis MG, McMahon FJ, Chase GA, Simpson SG, Ross CA, DePaulo JR Jr (1993) Anticipation in bipolar affective disorder [see comments]. Am J Hum Genet 53: 385–390

Mendlewicz J, Fleiss, JL (1974) Linkage studies with X-chromosome markers in bipolar (manic-depressive) illness. Biol Psychiatry 9: 261–294

Mendlewicz J, Fleiss JL, Fieve RR (1972) Evidence for X-linkage in the transmission of manic-depressive illness. JAMA 222: 1624–1627

Mendlewicz J, Simon P, Sevy S et al. (1987) Polymorphic DNA marker on X chromosome and manic-depression. Lancet 1 (8544): 1230–1232

Mendlewicz J, Leboyer M, De Bruyn A, Malafosse A, Sevy S, Hirsch D, Van Broeckhoven C, Mallet J (1991) Absence of linkage between chromosome 11p15 markers and manic-depressive illness in a Belgian pedigree. Am J Psychiatry 148: 1683–1687

Mitchell P, Waters B, Morrison N, Shine J, Donald J, Eisman J (1991) Close linkage of bipolar disorder to chromosome 11 markers is excluded in two large Australian pedigrees. J Affective Disord 21: 23–32

Mitchell P, Selbie L, Waters B, Donald J, Vivero C, Tully M, Shine J (1992) Exclusion of close linkage of bipolar disorder to dopamine D_1 and D_2 receptor gene markers. J Affective Disord 25: 1–11

Mitchell P, Waters B, Vivero C, Le F, Donald J, Tully M, Campedelli K, Lannfelt L, Sokoloff P, Shine J (1993) Exclusion of close linkage of bipolar disorder to the dopamine D_3 receptor gene in nine Australian pedigrees. J Affective Disord 27: 213–224

Nanko S, Kobayashi M, Gamou S, Kudoh J, Shimizu N, Takazawa N, Kazamatsuri H, Furusho T (1991) Linkage analysis of affective disorder using DNA markers on chromosomes 11 and X. Jpn J Psychiatry Neurol 45: 53–56

Nothen MM, Erdmann J, Korner J, Lanczik M, Fritze J, Fimmers R, Grandy DK, O'Dowd B, Propping P (1992) Lack of association between dopamine D_1 and D_2 receptor genes and bipolar affective disorder. Am J Psychiatry 149: 199–201
Nurnberger JI Jr, Goldin LR, Gershon ES (1994) Genetics of psychiatric disorders. In: Winokur G, Clayton PJ (eds) The medical basis of psychiatry. Saunders, Philadelphia, pp 459–492
Pakstis AJ, Kidd JR, Castiglione CM, Kidd KK (1991) Status of the search for a major genetic locus for affective disorder in the Old Order Amish. Hum Genet 87: 475–483
Pauls DL, Gerhard DS, Lacy LG, Hostetter AM, Allen CR, Bland SD, LaBuda MC, Egeland JA (1991) Linkage of bipolar affective disorders to markers on chromosome 11p is excluded in a second lateral extension of Amish pedigree 110. Genomics 11: 730–736
Pekkarinen P, Bredbacka PE, Terwilliger J, Hovatta I, Lonnqvist J, Peltonen L (1994) Evidence for a susceptibility locus for manic-depressive disorder in Xq26 (Abstr.) Am J Hum Genet 55: A133
Reich T, Clayton PJ, Winokur G (1969) Family history studies: the genetics of mania. Am J Psychiatry 125: 1358–1368
Rietschel M, Nothen MM, Lannfelt L, Sokoloff P, Schwartz JC, Lanczik M, Fritze J, Cichon S, Fimmers R, Korner J (1993) A serine to glycine substitution at position 9 in the extracellular N-terminal part of the dopamine D_3 receptor protein: no role in the genetic predisposition to bipolar affective disorder. Psychiatry Res 46: 253–259
Risch N (1990) Linkage strategies for genetically complex traits. I. Multilocus models. Am J Hum Genet 46: 222–228
Schaid DJ, Sommer SS (1993) Genotype relative risks: methods for design and analysis of candidate-gene association studies. Am J Hum Genet 53: 1114–1126
Shaikh S, Ball D, Craddock N, Castle D, Hunt N, Mant R, Owen M, Collier D, Gill M (1993) The dopamine D_3 receptor gene: no association with bipolar affective disorder. J Med Genet 30: 308–309
Sidenberg DG, King N, Kennedy JL (1994) Analysis of new D_4 dopamine receptor (DRD4) coding region variants and TH microsatellite in the Old Order Amish family (OOA110). Psychiatr Genet 4: 95–99
Simon GE, von Korff M (1992) Reevaluation of secular trends in depression rates. Am J Epidemiol 135: 1411–1422
Stine OC, DePaulo JR (1994) The Dana Foundation bipolar study: chromosome 18 (Abstr.). ACNP Annual Meeting Satellite, Dec 11, 1994 (Abstract)
Straub RE, Lehner T, Luo Y, Loth JE, Shao W, Sharpe L, Alexander JR, Das K, Simon R, Fieve RR, Lerer B, Endicott J, Ott J, Gilliam TC, Baron M (1994) A possible vulnerability locus for bipolar affective disorder on chromosome 21q22.3. Nature Genet 8: 291–296
Suarez BK, Rice JP, Reich T (1978) The generalized sib pair IBD distribution: its use in the detection of linkage. Ann Hum Genet 42: 87–94
Suarez BK, Hampe CL, VanEerdewegh PV (1994) Problems of replicating linkage claims in psychiatry. In: Gershon ES, Cloninger CR (eds) Genetic approaches to mental disorders. American Psychiatric, Washington, pp 23–46
Weeks DE, Lange K (1988) The affected-pedigree-member method of linkage analysis. Am J Hum Genet 42: 315–326

Targeting the Action of Antidepressant Drugs on Second-Messenger Systems

G. Racagni, M. Popoli, S. Mori, N. Brunello, and J. Perez

Introduction

Studies of the function of neuronal systems in depression have shifted in the last years from investigations of neurotransmitter turnover/metabolism and receptor binding to more molecular assessment strategies such as intracellular targets beyond the receptors. G proteins (Lesch et al. 1991; Ozawa and Rasenick 1991), second messengers, [cyclic adenosine monophosphate (cAMP) and cyclic guanosine monophosphate (cGMP)] (Vetulani and Sulser 1975; Rao et al. 1990; Varrault et al. 1991), protein kinases (Nestler et al. 1989; Perez et al. 1989; Racagni et al. 1992), and transcriptional/posttranscriptional variables and gene expression (Nestler et al. 1990; Brady et al. 1991) have been investigated in the action of antidepressant drugs.

These studies have clearly pointed out that signal transduction pathways could represent an important target to explain not only the molecular mechanisms of antidepressant action, but also the etiology/pathophysiology of affective disorders. Stimulation of different signaling cascades results in activation of protein kinases. In this report the role of cAMP dependent protein kinase (cAMP-PK) and calcium/calmodulin-dependent protein kinase II (CaMK II) will be discussed in the action of antidepressants.

Postsynaptic cAMP-Dependent Protein Kinase in the Action of Antidepressants

Within the cell, cAMP-dependent protein kinase (cAMP-PK) is a central component of cAMP signaling, since with very few exceptions all known cAMP-dependent effects are mediated through the activation of this enzyme. In the absence of cAMP, the enzyme exists as an inactive tetrameric complex, composed of two catalytic (C) and a regulatory (R) subunit dimer which represents the receptor for cAMP. Activation occurs by cAMP binding to regulatory subunits, which promote dissociation of the complex and the release of the free and active catalytic subunits. Once released from the holoenzyme state, C moieties are able to phosphorylate specific substrate proteins which in turn regulate a variety of cellular functions such as receptor desensitization, ion channel sensitivity, cytoskeleton organization, and gene expression.

Accordingly, the regulation of cAMP receptors represents a fundamental step in signal transduction and a possible target for drugs that modify neurotransmission such as antidepressants. We have shown that 10 days of treatment with desmethylimipramine (DMI), a tricyclic antidepressant, increased the amount of a protein band in rat cerebral cortex that, for its biochemical properties, appears to be the R subunit of cAMP-PK. Further characterization of this result was obtained by a combination of sodium dodecyl sulfate polyacrylamide gel electophoresis SDS-PAGE, photoaffinity labeling with $8N_3$ [^{32}P]cAMP, and autoradiography. DMI given for 10 days enhanced the covalent binding of [^{32}P]cAMP to the R subunit in the soluble fraction of rat cerebral cortex. Moreover, we have demonstrated that other antidepressants such as fluoxetine and (+)- oxaprotiline, which specifically blocks serotonin and norepinephrine uptake, were also able to affect the cAMP binding to R subunits after 10 days of treatment. In addition, we have found that moclobemide, a reversible monoamine oxidase (MAO). A inhibitor enhanced the covalent binding of [^{32}P]cAMP to R subunits in the soluble fraction of rat cerebral cortex after 20 days of treatment.

Recent evidence obtained in our laboratory indicates that at least in rat cerebral cortex, cAMP-PK type II is associated with microtubules through the binding of R subunits to specific microtubule-associated proteins (Perez et al. 1993). These findings suggest that within the cell, microtubules could play an important role in the modulation of the intracellular signal transduction processes.

Interestingly, after 10 days of treatment, DMI, fluoxetine, and (+)- oxaprotiline were able to increase the covalent binding of [^{32}P]cAMP into the 52-kDa cAMP receptor associated with the rat cerebrocortical microtubule fraction.

To evaluate whether the increase in the amount of R subunit could have been elicited by a modification in the transcriptional activity, we have performed in situ hybridization experiments. Under these conditions chronic administration of DMI was unable to affect the expression of mRNA for R subunits. Therefore, we hypothesize that translational changes of the enzyme might be involved in these modifications. In conclusion these results strongly suggest that cAMP protein kinase could be an intracellular target for the action of antidepressant drugs.

Presynaptic Calcium/Calmodulin-Dependent Protein Kinase II, Modulation of Transmitter Release, and the Action of Psychotropic Drugs

Calcium/calmodulin-dependent protein kinase II (CaMK II), also referred to as multifunctional CaM kinase, is a ubiquitary kinase mediating a great variety of cellular responses to calcium (Hanson and Schulman 1992). CaMK II is 20- to 50-fold more concentrated in brain than in non nervous tissues, and is enriched in cortical stuctures, particularly in the hippocampus (2% of total protein). The kinase is concentrated at both sides of the synapse inside presynaptic terminals and in postsynaptic densities (PSD), where it constitutes between 20% and 40% of total protein (Fig. 1) (Hanson and Schulman 1992).

Several lines of evidence have demonstrated that CaMK II is involved in the modulation of transmitter release from the presynapse and in various forms of synaptic plasticity, including long-term potentiation (LTP), a cellular model of learning and memory (Nichols et al. 1990; Silva et al. 1992; Fukunaga et al. 1995). In the presynapse CaMK II phosphorylates several substrates, the two best-known being synapsin I and synaptotagmin (Greengard et al. 1993; Popoli 1993a), two

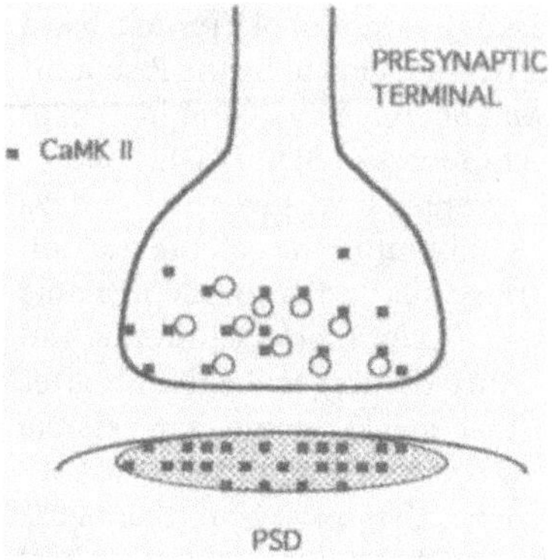

Fig. 1. Schematic diagram of calcium/calmodulin-dependent protein kinase II (*CaMK II, solid squares*), concentrations at both sides of the synapse – inside presynaptic terminals and in postsynaptic densities (*PSD*)

proteins of synaptic vesicles. In the postsynaptic compartment the kinase is known to phosphorylate several proteins, induding MAP2 and, in PSD, the non-*N*-methyl-*D*-aspartate (NMDA)glutamate receptor subunit GluR1 (Hanson and Schulman 1992; McGlade-McCulloh et al. 1993). Hereafter we will be concerned only with presynaptic aspects of CaMK II function.

The presynaptic kinase autophosphorylates following depolarization of synaptic terminals, becoming calcium-independent (autonomous) (Gorelick et al. 1988): introduction of this autonomous kinase into isolated synaptic terminals stimulates transmitter release (Nichols et al. 1990). Several substrates of CaMK II, all proteins of synaptic vesicles, could be involved in this effect. The best characterized among them is synapsin I. This protein anchors synaptic vesicles in the reserve pool to the actin-based cytoskeleton. Phosphorylation on two residues, promoted by CaMK II, releases synapsin and the vesicles from the cytoskeleton, increasing the number of vesicles available for exocytosis (Greengard et al. 1993). Another major substrate of the kinase is synaptotagmin, a protein which participates in the multimolecular complex regulating docking and fusion of the vesicles, and is a putative Ca^{2+} receptor in the molecular machinery controlling exocytosis. The role of phosphorylation in the control of its activity is much less known (Popoli 1993b).

Although in recent years a great deal of work was carried out on the molecular machinery regulating presynaptic release, very little is known about the plastic changes induced by psychotropic drugs in the process of transmitter release. Some of the drugs used in the therapy of affective disorders appear to have a presynaptic effect. It was shown that long-term treatment with various antidepressant drugs causes an enhancement of neurotransmission in a number of pathways, including the neurons projecting from the raphe nuclei to the hippocampus (Blier and de Montigny 1994). Whereas some drugs (i.e., tricyclics) work by sentizing 5-hydroxytryptamine (5-HT) postsynaptic receptors on hippocampal pyramidal cells, others, like selective serotonin reuptake inhibitors (SSRI), seem to promote a desensitization of 5-HT presynaptic receptors and a consequent increase in 5-HT release (Blier and Bouchard 1994).

To investigate whether CaMK II and the release molecular machinery are involved in this drug-induced plasticity, subcellular fractions enriched in synaptic vesices, synaptic cytosol and synaptosomal membranes were prepared from the hippocampus and cortex of animals after long-term treatment with two SSRI (paroxetine and fluvoxamine) and a mixed 5-HT and noradrenaline (NA) reuptake inhibitor (venlafaxine). All fractions were subjected to endogenous Ca^{2+}/CaM-dependent phosphorylation (Popoli 1993a), phosphoproteins were separated by denaturing electrophoresis, and phosphate incorporation into individual bands was quantitated by computer-assisted densitometry. As shown in Fig. 2, the extent of autophosphorylation of α-CaMK II (the predominant isoform in the forebrain) was greatly increased in hippocampal synaptic vesicles compared to the control animals. A roughly equivalent change was induced by the three drugs used (between 110 % and 145 %). In the same samples, phosphorylation of the bands containing the two major substrates, synapsin I and synaptotagmin, was also increased. A similar kinase autophosphorylation increase was observed in the soluble (synaptic cytosol) population of the enzyme. No significant change was detected either in the kinase or in the substrates in synaptosomal membranes. As synaptosomal membranes contain mostly postsynaptic CaMK II, associated with the postsynaptic membrane attached to the synaptosomes (Rostas and Dunkley 1992), the change in the Ca^{2+}/CaM-stimulated phosphorylation system appears to be restricted to the presynaptic compartment. No change was detected in all fractions prepared from total cortex (not shown). As increased transmitter release after SSRI treatment, was measured in other areas besides the hippocampus (hypothalamus, frontal cortex), it is conceivable that the effect in selected areas is diluted when presynaptic fractions are prepared from total cortex.

Interestingly, in synaptic vesicles from the hippocampus (Fig. 2) phosphorylation of synapsin I increased only moderately with two of the drugs (+28 %), reaching significance only with paroxetine (+70 %). On the contrary, phosphorylation increase in the synaptotagmin band was comparable to that of CaMK II (110 – 160 %) and significant with all the drugs. As the β-isoform of CaMK II (3 to 4 times less abundant than α-CaMK II) comigrates with synaptotagmin, its presence could alter the measurement of synaptotagmin phosphorylation.

To avoid interference in the measure it is necessary to immunoprecipitate the protein and measure phosphate incorporation into the isolated protein. Preliminary experiments showed that synaptotagmin phosphorylation increased between 85 % and 110 %, confirming a remarkable, significant increase. Synapsin and synaptotagmin conceivably control different steps of the synaptic vesicle cycle, with the former regulating availability of the vesicles and the latter presumably being involved in a priming step which enables already docked vesicles to respond to the calcium influx. Preferential phosphorylation of one of the CaMK II substrates may give useful suggestions as to the molecular steps involved in the action of drugs on neurotransmitter release.

As for the CaMK II autophosphorylation increase, it was demonstrated that it is associated with an increase in the Ca^{2+}/CaM-dependent activity of the kinase in the presynapse (Popoli et al. 1995). No changes in activity or autophosphorylation of presynaptic CaMK II were induced by acute treatment. In all cases the increase was due to greater phosphate incorporation, and not to neosynthesis or translocation of the kinase. Therefore it appears that a long-lasting modification was induced in presynaptic CaMK II activity in the hippocampus of animals chronically treated with 5-HT reuptake blockers, possibly through a cascade of events starting with desensitization of presynaptic 5-HT receptors.

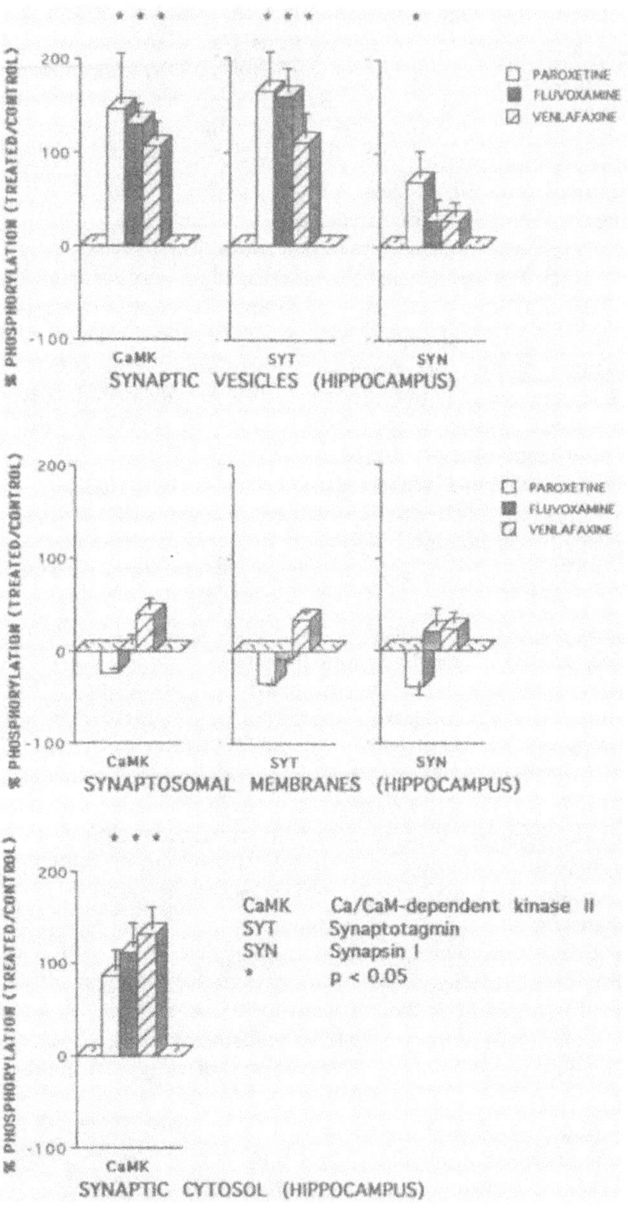

Fig. 2. Percentage of phosphorylation ratio (treated vs control) of CaMKII, synaptotagmin, and synapsin I after long-term treatment with selective serotonin reuptake inhibitors (SSRI) (paroxetine or fluvoxamine) and venlafaxine. In the presence of Ca^{2+}/calmodulin, 10–20 μg protein/fraction was subjected to endogenous phosphorylation with [γ-^{32}P]ATP. Proteins were separated by denaturing electrophoresis and autoradiographies obtained. Phosphate incorporation was measured using charge-coupled device (CCD) camera images of autoradiograhies and a computer program for image analysis (Image 1.47, National Institute of Health)

Long-lasting modifications of CaMK II were described in physiological events, like LTP, and pathological ones, like ischemia, glutamate-induced neurotoxicity, and seizures (Hanson and Schulman 1992). In one ischemia model it was shown that the change is due to a posttranslational modification which decreases the kinase affinity for ATP (Churn et al 1992).

In a recent report (Meshul and Tan 1994) it was shown that chronic haloperidol treatment induces a large increase of CaMK II activity in synaptic membranes in the striatum. This finding was associated with a decrease of glutamate immunoreactivity inside presynaptic terminals, interpreted by the authors as a consequence of increased glutamate release, previously found following treatment with dopamine D_2-receptor selective blockers. The authors suggest that chronic blockade of presynaptic D_2 receptors results in an increase of transmitter release in the corticostriatal tract. Even though no attempt was made to distinguish between pre- and postsynaptic CaMK II, it was argued that at least part of the activity increase is due to the presynaptic kinase, which increases phosphorylation of proteins participating in the release machinery. This eventually leads to an increase in transmitter release. The report proposes that this process may be one of the sites of action of antipsychotic drugs, being involved in the relieving of the psychosis as well as in the extrapyramidal side effects often observed in treated patients.

It is remarkable that drugs as diverse as 5-HT reuptake blockers and D_2 – receptor blockers may exert some of their actions by working on the presynaptic release apparatus. It is tempting to speculate that this mechanism of action could be common to several different drugs acting on presynaptic terminals in different brain areas. Whenever the drugs cause, directly or indirectly, desensitization or blockade of presynaptic receptors which have a tonic inhibitory action on transmitter release, stimulation of CaMK II and of effectors in the release apparatus may result. We think this could be a useful working hypothesis in the investigation of drug-induced neural plasticity as well as in the study of the pathophysiology of neuropsychiatric disorders.

Conclusions

In summary, our data seem to support the existence of intracellular targets in the action of antidepressant drugs. Activation of specific protein kinases could represent an important step in a cascade of signaling pathways which transfer messages from the membrane receptors to the nucleus.

Antidepressants increase the synaptic concentrations of neurotransmitters after acute administration; consequently pre- and post-synaptic receptors coupled second messenger systems are activated.

CaMK II and cAMP-PK are two kinases which could play an important role in the long-term administration of antidepressants. In fact, their activation promotes fundamental functional changes in the substrate proteins both at presynaptic and postsynaptic level. These modifications could explain the delay in the action of these drugs. Therefore, studies on the involvement of protein phosphorylation might provide greater knowledge about the molecular basis of affective disorders and provide new insights for designing novel antidepressant drugs.

References

Blier P, de Montigny C (1994) Trends Pharmacol Sci 15: 220–225
Blier P, Bouchard C (1994) Br J Pharmacol 113: 485–495
Brady SL, Whitfield HJ, Fox RJ, Gold PW, Herkenham M (1991) J Clin Invest 87: 831–837
Churn SB, Taft WC, Billingsley MS, Sankaran B, De Lorenzo RJ (1992) J Neurochem 59: 1221–1232
Fukunaga K, Muller D, Miyamoto E (1995) J Biol Chem 270: 6119–6124
Gorelick FS, Wang JKT, Lai Y, Nairn A, Greengard P (1988) J Biol Chem 263: 17209–17212
Greengard P, Valtorta F, Czernik AJ, Benfenati F (1993) Science 259: 780–785
Hanson PI, Schulman H (1992) Annu Rev Biochem 61: 559–601
Lesch KP, Aulakh CS, Tolliver TJ, Hill JL, Murphy DL (1991) Eur J Pharmacol 207: 361–364
McGlade-McCulloh E, Yamamoto H, Tan S, Brickey D, Soderling T (1993) Nature 362: 640–642
Meshul CK, Tan S (1994) Synapse 18: 205–217
Nestler EJ, Terwillinger RZ, Duman RS (1989) Eur J Pharmacol 53: 1644–1647
Nestler EJ, McMahon A, Sabban EL, Tallman JF, Duman RS (1990) Proc Natl Acad Sci USA 87: 7522–7526
Nichols RA, Sihra TS, Czernik AJ, Nairn AC, Greengard P (1990) Nature 343: 647–651
Ozawa H, Rasenick MM (1991) Mol Pharmacol 36: 803–808
Perez J, Tinelli D, Brunello N, Racagni G (1989) Eur J Pharmacol 172: 305–316
Perez J, Tinelli D, Cagnoli C, Pecin P, Brunello N, Racagni G (1993) Brain Res 602: 77–83
Popoli M (1993a) FEBS Lett 317: 85–88
Popoli (1993b) Neuroscience 54: 323–328
Popoli M, Vocaturo C, Perez J, Smeraldi E, Racagni G (1995) Mol Pharmacol 48 (in press)
Racagni G, Brunello N, Tinelli D, Perez J (1992) Pharamcopsychiatry 25: 51–55
Rao TS, Cler JA, Mick SJ, Ragan DM, Lanthorn TH, Contreras PC, Iyengar S, Wood PL (1990) Neuropharmacology 29 (12): 1199–1204
Rostas JAP, Dunkley P (1992) J Neurochem 59: 1191–1202
Silva AJ, Stevens CF, Tonegawa S, Wang Y (1992) Science 257: 201–206
Varrault A, Leviel V, Backaert J (1991) J Pharmacol Exp Ther 257 (1): 433–438
Vetulani J, Sulser F (1975) Nature 297: 495–496

New Concepts of Schizophrenia Derived from Epidemiological Research

H. Häfner

Introduction

When I received the honourable invitation as one of the two indigenous speakers to present a lecture in honour of my friend Hanns Hippius for his 70th birthday at this holy place, I got the uneasy feeling that something remarkable was expected of me. Also worried by the fact that I had been included with an ambitious epidemiological topic in a purely psychopharmacological programme, I realised that I owed my friend at least a brief glimpse of the biological depths from the epidemiological surface – the more so since our great forerunner Sigmund Freud had tried in vain to fish for the causes of schizophrenia with his psychoanalytic hook, finding merely his own mirror image staring at him from the depths.

Cautious as I am, I shall concentrate on simple questions: on the influence of gender on the onset of schizophrenia and the reasons for this and, in further analyses, on the onset of schizophrenia and its impeding effects on individual social development. I shall begin with previously published results from our ABC schizophrenia study, which was launched in 1987 and is scheduled to be completed in 1998, and then present some new findings.

What Kind of Disease is Schizophrenia?

The WHO *Determinants of Outcome* study (Jablensky et al. 1992) showed that age-standardised incidence rates, when based on a restrictive and precise definition of schizophrenia, hardly vary at all across countries and cultures. This exceptional epidemiological finding, which has been observed in the same form with only very few syndromes of heterogeneous origin such as Alzheimer's disease or moderately severe and severe mental retardation, allows only a negative conclusion to be drawn, namely, that culture or the social system does not have any great aetiological bearing on the risk of morbidity.

The fact that first admissions for schizophrenia have consistently been found to cluster in the low socioeconomic class and the finding that the incidence of schizophrenia can be associated with various spatial factors in small geographical areas have equally failed to provide promising clues to the aetiology of the disorder. The causal explanation of the social gradient of schizophrenia was recently refuted by Dohrenwend et al. (1992) in a methodologically elegant population study in Israel. The social selection processes capable of producing uneven socioeconomic and spatial distributions of schizophrenia on a small geographical scale are obviously accounted for by premorbid functional deficits or early consequences of the disorder. But uneven distributions across socioeconomic strata and small areas do not necessarily contradict an even distribution of the risk of morbidity across total populations, because the effects of internal selection processes should actually be counterbalanced in large and comprehensive populations such as nations.

Equal incidence rates in different populations, climates, and societies cannot be explained by one single disease cause, because disease causes usually vary geographically with environmental and genetic factors. There are presumably several causes which level out the effects of a single risk factor that shows variation. These first conclusions already suggest that schizophrenia presumably represents a syndrome that has a multiple aetiology, but is encountered in all human cultures in almost the same form and at approximately the same frequency.

Sex Difference in Age at First Onset

Epidemiology can produce clues to aetiological or pathogenetic factors if it reveals consistent deviations from expected values in the distribution pattern of a risk of morbidity. There is indeed an epidemiological finding, both exceptional and stable, that has not yet been explained conclusively: Kraepelin, one of Professor Hippius's predecessors on the chair for psychiatry in Munich, reported in 1909 that women, compared with men, tended to be several years older on average when hospitalised for the first time for dementia praecox. Since then the sex difference has been confirmed in more than 50 studies (Strömgren 1935; Lindelius 1970; Angermeyer and Kühn 1988). We undertook our study with the aim of clarifying the causes of this difference by adopting a systematic research strategy.

In a total of nine substudies we first replicated the finding together with Munk-Jørgensen and the late Erik Strömgren on data from the Danish and the Mannheim case registers. Age-standardised, population-based rates for various diagnostic definitions were calculated, and highly significant differences ranging from 4 to 5 years were found (Table 1). Alternative explanations, such as a milder early symptomatology in women, or a lower social tolerance of abnormal behaviour – prompting earlier hospitalisation – in men, were excluded. The next step led us to direct testing of the hypothesis that a sex difference in age at onset may explain the difference in age at first admission. For this purpose we construed, on the basis of internationally approved instruments, a standardised interview called "Instrument for the Retrospective Assessment of the Onset of Schizophrenia" (IRAOS), for a retrospective assessment of symptomatology and social development by means of a time grid extending from onset to first admission (Häfner et al. 1990, 1992). With this instrument, information is obtained from three independent sources: the patient, a key informant and available case notes or medical records. Its reliability ranged from satisfactory to good.

Table 1. Mean age (in years) at first admission for a broad or restricted definition of schizophrenia in Denmark (1976) and Mannheim (1978–80)

	Broad definition		Restricted definition	
	DK (n = 1169)	MA (n = 336)	DK	MA
Males	34.8	33.1	32.8	32.5
Age difference	5.4	4.8	4.9	3.9
Females	40.2	37.9	37.7	36.4

DK, Denmark; MA, Mannheim. On the basis of population-based rates per 5-year age groups. $p \leq .001$. (From Häfner et al. 1989.)

Sample

Data were collected on all patients who, over a 2-year period, had been admitted for the first time on the basis of a broad diagnostic definition of schizophrenia or nonaffective functional psychosis to any of the ten psychiatric hospitals and units serving a population of 1.5 million. Figure 1 depicts the cities of Heidelberg and

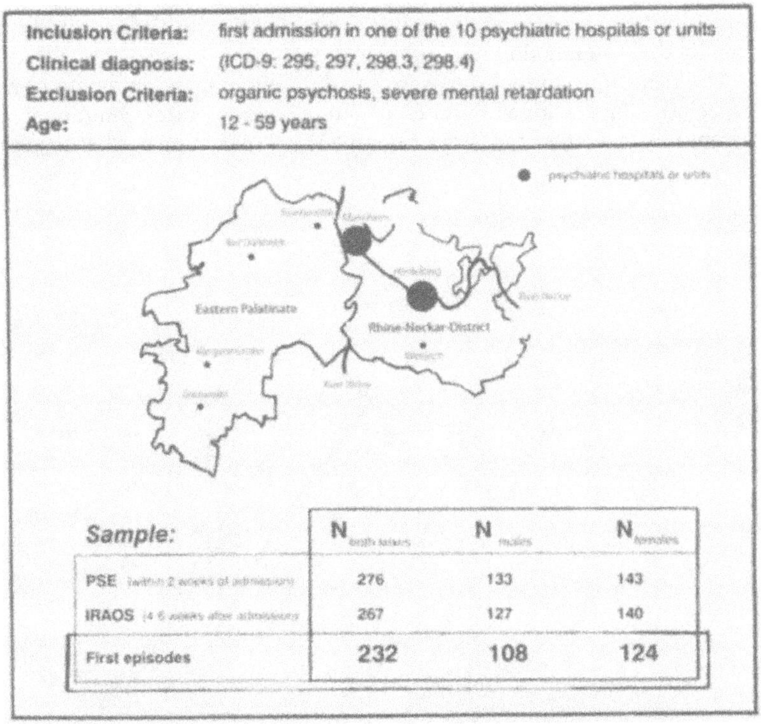

Fig. 1. ABC first-episode sample showing catchment area of Rhine-Neckar district and eastern Palatinate with ca. 1.5 million inhabitants. *PSE*, Present State Examination; *IRAOS*, Instrument for the Retrospective Assessment of the Onset of Schizophrenia. (From Häfner et al. 1995)

Mannheim with their surrounding regions and the eastern Palatinate and gives the sizes of the study samples. Of the total of 276 cases assigned to PSE-CATEGO (a computer programme for analyzing PSE data; the acronym is derived from "to categorize") diagnoses, 232 (84%) were first episodes.

Mean age at first onset was compared between the sexes for various definitions of onset: first-ever sign of mental disorder, first negative symptom, first positive symptom, maximum of positive symptoms (our definition of the climax of the first episode), and, finally, first admission. Significant differences ranging from 3 to 4 years emerged (Fig. 2). By courtesy of Dr. Norman Sartorius the finding was tested for transnational stability on pooled data from the 12 centres in 10 countries participating in the WHO *Determinants of Outcome* study, and a highly significant mean age difference of 3.4 years was found (Hambrecht et al. 1992).

To look for indications of sex-related aetiological factors we compared the lifetime risk for men and women. Figure 3 shows cumulative, population-based incidence rates for males and females in successive 5-year age groups. At the end of the main age-of-risk range, that is, at age 59, men showed a total rate of 13.21 and women, 13.14. When a restrictive diagnostic definition was applied, no essential changes occurred. Since the cumulative incidence calculated across the relevant risk period for schizophrenia is a good indicator of the lifetime risk, the obvious conclusion from this finding is that the lifetime risk or the mean liability to develop schizophrenia is equal in men and women. Men just consume their risk of morbidity clearly more rapidly than women do.

The next thing to look for were sex differences in symptomatology and course, especially since a great number of studies report more emotional and positive symptoms in women and more negative symptoms in men. The very few epidemio-

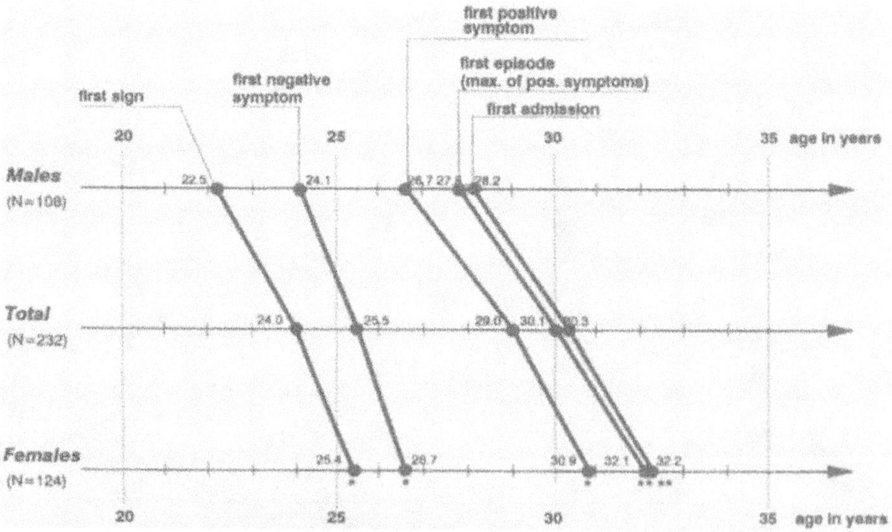

Fig. 2. Mean age values at five definitions of onset until first admission. First-episode sample of schizophrenia, broad definition ($n = 232$); $^{*}p \leq 0.05$; $^{**}p \leq 0.01$

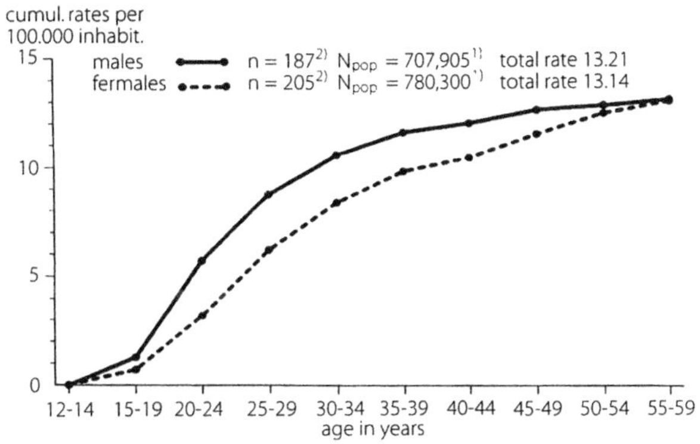

Fig. 3. Cumulative incidence rates for schizophrenia, broad definition (ICD-9 295, 297, 298.3, and 298.4). [1)] N_{pop}, total population; [2)] *n*, number of patients in 2 years. Source of data: a representative first-admission sample (1987/89) *n*=392; catchment area: Mannheim, Heidelberg, Rhine-Neckar district, eastern Palatinate. (From Häfner et al. 1991b)

logical follow-up studies (Biehl et al. 1986; Salokangas et al. 1987; Tsuang and Fleming 1987; Shepherd et al. 1989) have revealed few or no differences in early symptomatology, but a consistently poorer social outcome in men at least in the first 5 years after first admission.

We defined type of onset or early course according to the interval between the appearance of the first-ever symptom and first admission and distinguished between an acute type of onset with a length of up to 4 weeks, a subacute type of 4 weeks to 1 year and a chronic type of more than 1 year. As Table 2 shows, no significant differences emerged. With a difference as small as 65%–70%, we were unable to demonstrate a predominance of the chronic or insidious type of onset among men. Noteworthy is that 68% of the cases had begun with a prephase of more than 1 year.

We divided early course into a prodromal phase, extending until the appearance of the first positive symptom, and a psychotic prephase, ending with the climax of the first episode, and found that 73% of the first-episode cases had developed nonspecific or negative symptoms before the psychotic episode started. We then distinguished between the three traditional symptom categories of positive, negative

Table 2. Onset of schizophrenia

	ABC first-episode sample		
	Total *n* = 232	Males *n* = 108	Females *n* = 124
Type of onset			
Acute (≤ 1 month)	18%	19%	17%
Subacute (> 1 month ≤ 1 year)	15%	11%	18%
Insidious or chronic (> 1 year)	68%	70%	65%
*Type of first symptoms**			
Negative or nonspecific	73%	70%	76%
Positive	7%	7%	6%
Both	20%	22%	19%

ABC, author's schizophrenia study.
* No significant gender differences in the variables listed.

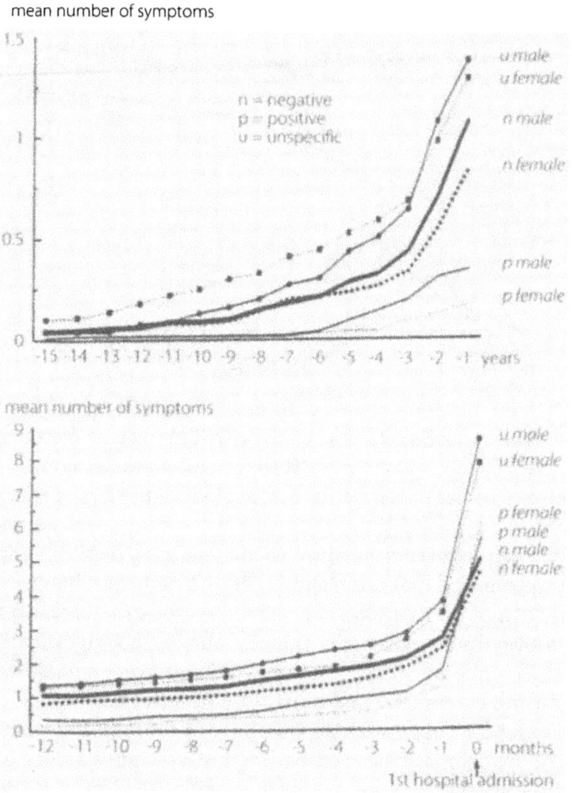

Fig. 4. Cumulative numbers of positive, negative and unspecific symptoms of onset of schizophrenia until first hospital admission for schizophrenia (males = 108; females = 124). (From Häfner et al. 1995)

Table 3. Rank order of the five most frequent initial symptoms of schizophrenia

	ABC study: first-episode sample					
	Total (n = 232)		Males (n = 108)		Females (n = 124)	
	n	%	n	%	n	%
1. Concentration and subjective thought disorder	50	22	28	26	22	18
2. Lack of energy, slowness	45	19	19	18	26	21
3. Suspiciousness, social withdrawal	44	19	23	21	21	17
4. Overall slowing down	37	16	15	14	22	18
5. Anxiety	32	14	16	15	16	13

No significant gender differences.
Analysis based on phase model. Symptoms taken into account for operationalization of onset; nonspecific symptoms only if continuously present until index admission;
negative symptoms only if continuous or recurrent;
positive symptoms in any case, even if they occurred only once.

and nonspecific symptoms and depicted their accumulation year by year until 1 year before first admission and, because of the very steep increase, in the last year month by month (Fig. 4). Again, no substantial sex differences became visible.

The five most frequent initial symptoms of schizophrenia, too, did not differ between the sexes (Table 3). We then compared males and females with respect to all 272 items indicating symptoms, functional impairment or social disability and assessed by the Present State Examination (PSE), Scale for the Assessment of Negative Symptoms (SANS), Psychological Impairments Rating Schedule (PIRS) and Disability Assessment Schedule (DAS). None of the positive core symptoms and none of the negative symptoms showed significant sex differences. In Table 4 those 18 items that continued to show significant differences after an internal cross-validation are arranged into three groups according to their presumed closeness to the disease process. In females, particularly at a young age, sexual delusions and delusions of pregnancy and guilt predominate. It is very likely that theses delusions do not represent expressions of the illness, but rather sex-specific fantasies and forms of coping with the disorder. It is equally difficult to interpret the long list of 11 behavioural items, all of which are socially negative, that we found to predominate in schizophrenic men, and of the socially positive overcompliance, which we found to be more frequent in women, as direct expressions of the psychosis. Population studies have in fact revealed that men in the prime period of risk for schizophrenia, that is, between 15 and 25 years of age, show considerably higher rates of dissocial and partly also asocial and criminal behaviour and substance abuse compared with women

Table 4. Significant gender differences validated by split-half test in 18 out of 272 items at first admission ($n = 276$)

		Positive ratings		p	Relative risk
		Males (%)	Females (%)	(chi²)	m : f
Positive symptoms					
PSE 86	Sexual delusions	3.8	14.8	**	0.26
PSE 85	Delusions of pregnancy	0.0	7.7	*	0
+ 1 further item					
Nonspecific symptoms					
CATEGO 7	Obsessional neurosis	43.6	30.1	*	1.45
PSE 44	Obsessional checking, repeating	25.2	14.9	*	1.69
PSE 88	Delusions of guilt	7.0	16.1	*	0.43
Behavioural items					
PIRS 72	Self-neglect	34.9	18.4	**	1.90
DAS 13	Social withdrawal	77.9	56.5	**	1.38
DAS 40	Lack of interest in job	69.4	34.3	**	2.02
+ 8 further items of socially negative behaviour significantly more frequent in males					
PIRS 85	Overcompliance	4.8	15.2	**	0.32

* $p \leq .05$.
** $p \leq .01$.

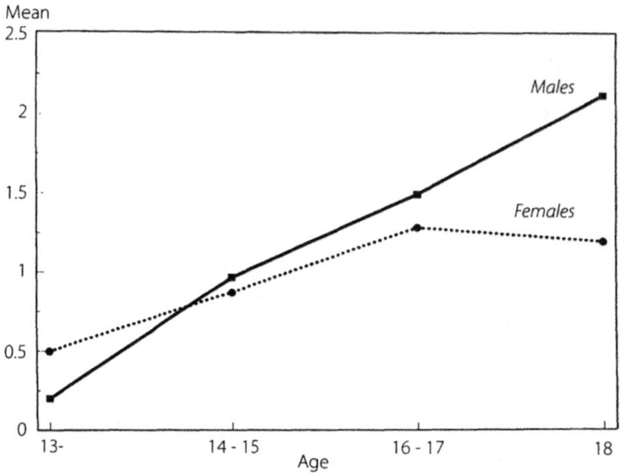

Fig. 5. Mean frequency of conduct disorders by age and sex. (From Choquet and Ledoux 1994)

(Fig. 5) (Choquet and Ledoux 1994). We therefore presume that the strong socially negative male behaviour and the weak preponderance of socially positive female behaviour represent forms of sex-specific illness behaviour that are triggered by the psychosis.

From the results that we have discussed so far, the astonishing conclusion must be drawn that illness variables, that is, type of onset and symptomatology, do not differ significantly between the sexes in early schizophrenia. The only essential differences of relevance to further course seem to be the lower age of onset and the predominance of socially negative illness behaviour in men.

Sex Differences in the Course of Schizophrenia

If the symptom-related early course is similar in men and women, how can the poorer social outcome of men in the first years after first admission be explained? In 77% of cases the prodromal phase began before age 30, that is, in the main period of social ascent in life, and in 41% before age 20 (Table 5). The initial symptoms and the

Table 5. Onset of schizophrenia

	ABC first-episode sample		
	Total $n = 232$	Males $n = 108$	Females $n = 124$
Age at onset of the earliest sign*			
< 10 years	4%	7%	2%
< 20 years	41%	46%	37%
< 30 years	77%	82%	73%

* No significant gender differences in the variable listed.

Table 6. Social role performance at the time of first sign of mental disorder

Age (in years)	Males $n = 108$ 22.5 %		Females $n = 124$ 25.4 %	Total $n = 232$ 24.0 %
School education (finished)	70		69	70
Occupational training	41	n. s.	38	39
Employment	37	*	52	45
Own accomodation	39	*	54	47
Marriage or stable partnership	28	**	52	41

t $p \leq 0.1$; * $p \leq 0.05$; ** $p \leq 0.01$; n. s., not significant

prephase of schizophrenia with a mean length of 5 years frequently involved signs of functional and cognitive impairment. We therefore presumed that the intrusion of schizophrenia into a phase of incomplete social and cognitive development might impede expected social ascent and probably also cognitive and personality development. We further hypothesised that, due to their younger age, men should be hit by onset at a lower level of social development. This should disrupt their further social ascent and result in a poorer social outcome.

To test this hypothesis we analysed which social roles were performed by men and women when the first sign of the disorder appeared. Table 6 shows five social roles, which we selected as examples and which are usually performed successively in the age range of 15 to 30 years. No significant differences between males and females appeared in terms of finished school education and occupational training. Significant differences of medium size were observed in employment and own income and a pronounced, highly significant difference in marriage or stable partnership. This confirmed our assumption that men are affected by the onset of schizophrenia at a lower level of social development than women.

The next question, to what extent schizophrenics fall short of the expected social development, required a case-control design. Previously published studies had compared the social achievement of schizophrenics with the socioeconomic statuses of their fathers or with social data of the general population. We compared a representative sample of 57 schizophrenics with 57 controls, matched for age and sex and drawn from the same population at risk, for level of social development at exactly the same age, determined by the patients' age at the appearance of the first sign of mental disorder, of first psychotic symptom and at first admission.

I shall present the results on only one of the social roles we studied, namely, marriage and stable partnership. Marrying 2.5 years later on average than women in the population at large, men showed significantly lower percentages of married-at-onset compared with women who were 3 years older (Fig. 6). In the following 6 years, "healthy" male controls reduced this difference by one-half. In contrast, in both male and female schizophrenics the downward trend continued across the total prephase. By the end of the prephase, the differences from controls had grown highly significant, with 17 % of schizophrenic males being married or in a stable partnership as compared to 60 % of the male controls. The corresponding figures for female schizophrenics and controls were 32 % and 80 %, respectively.

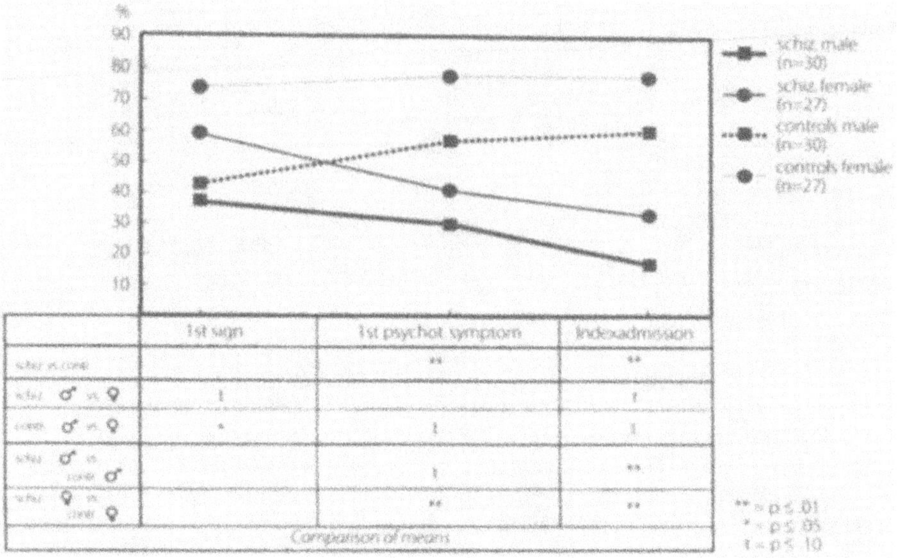

Fig. 6. Marriage or stable partnership

It is obvious that schizophrenics are most severely handicapped in establishing and maintaining highly intimate relationships involving little social distance. We concluded that schizophrenia starts to disrupt social development long before first admission, in some cases even leading to first steps of social decline. And men are more strongly affected than women, because they are hit by the illness at an earlier stage of their social development.

To test the hypothesis that the further social course of schizophrenia may be determined primarily by the level of social development at onset and illness behaviour in males rather than by disease-related variables, we assessed a representative sub-sample of 133 cases from our ABC sample at four waves over a 2-year period following first admission. Social disability, defined by a DAS score of ≥ 2, was chosen as the outcome variable. We presumed that male sex and a low age of onset should be associated with a low level of social development at onset, which again should increase social disability 2 years after first admission. An insidious onset and the severity of symptoms should also contribute to social disability. A global index of social deficits was made up of the following variables: unfinished occupational training, unemployment, lack of own income and lack of own accommodation. Stepwise logistic regression analyses were performed at three time points: (1) the appearance of the first sign of mental disorder, (2) the end of the prodromal phase, when the first positive symptom appeared and (3) the end of the psychotic prephase, that is, at first admission.

We found that when the first sign of mental disorder appeared it was not yet possible to predict social disability at 2 years after first admission to any significant degree. This result suggests that premorbid social deficits are not a strong predictor at least of this particular measure of social disability. On the other hand, the result

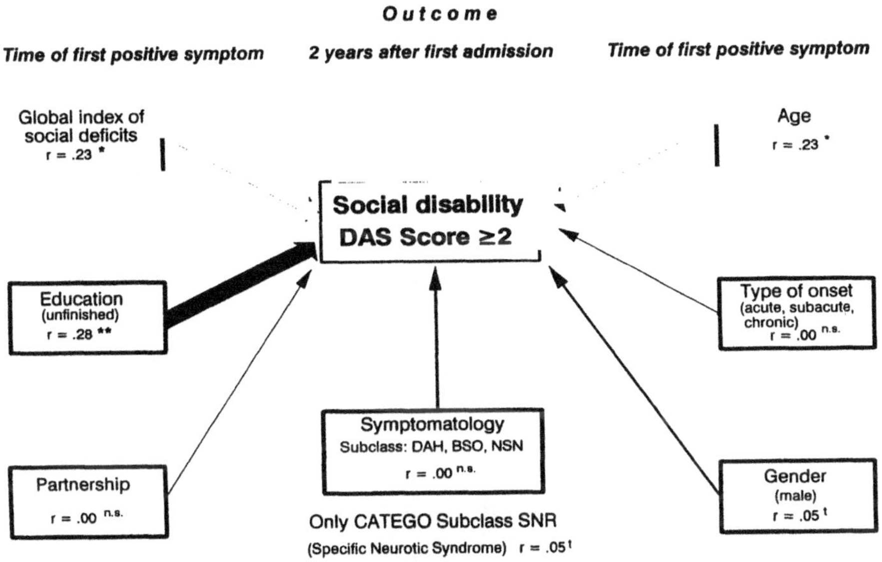

Fig. 7. Prediction model of social disability (correct overall classification 81%). *DAS*, Disability Assessment Schedule; *CATEGO*,; *DAH*, Delusions and Hallucinations; *BSO*, Behaviour, Speech and other Syndromes; *NSN*, Non-Specific Neurotic Syndrome; *SNR*, Specific Neurotic Syndrome; *r* partial correlation. (From Häfner et al. 1995)

might also reflect a generally rather low level of social development at this age. At the end of the prodromal phase, when the first psychotic symptom occurs, the model enabled us to predict social disability 2 years after first admission with an overall accuracy of 81% correct classifications. As shown in Fig. 7, neither type of onset nor symptomatology as assessed by the PSE – apart from CATEGO subclass Specific Neurotic Syndrome (SNR), which includes items of social behaviour – had any predictive power. In line with our hypothesis, the highest and significant partial correlations were obtained with unfinished school education, the global index of social deficits and age at onset of the first psychotic episode. Hence, we were able to show that the level of social development mediated by age at illness onset is by far the most important determinant of social disability at least in the first 2 years after first admission. In addition, male sex has an independent effect, which can probably be explained by the socially negative illness behaviour of young males.

Why Do Women Fall Ill with Schizophrenia Later than Men?

Now that we had established that age at onset plays a greater role than symptomatology and type of onset in determining social disadvantage in the early course of schizophrenia, we had to clarify why women fall ill 3 to 4 years later on average than men. Figure 8 gives the percentages of onset, defined by the first sign of

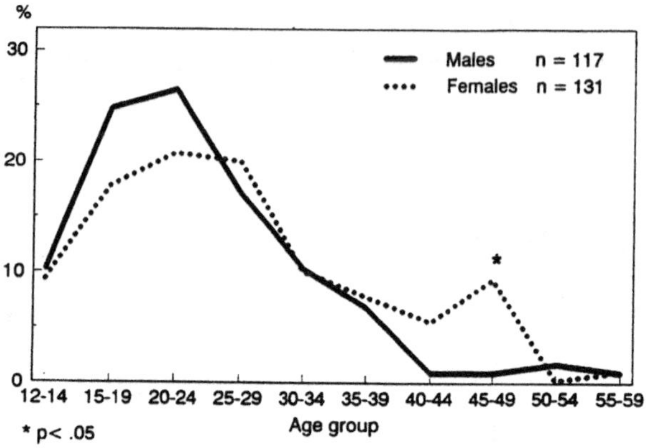

Fig. 8. Age distribution of onsets of schizophrenia (first-ever sign of mental disorder) for males and females (ICD 9-295, 297, 298.3, 298.4). ABC sample: Mannheim, Heidelberg, Rhine-Neckar district, eastern Palatinate. (From Häfner et al. 1995)

mental disorder, for 5-year age groups across the total age range up to 60 years. Males show a steep increase and an early peak followed by a steady decline. Females exhibit a slower increase, a lower first peak and, after a decline, a second peak at ages 45 to 49, which significantly deviates from the male trend in this age group.

This pattern of distribution of onsets across the female life cycle and the well-known neuroleptic-like effects of acute estradiol administration in animal experiments (Henn and McKinney 1987; Harrer 1987; DiPaolo and Falardeau 1985; Fields and Gordon 1982) prompted us to postulate that estrogen might delay onset in females by increasing the vulnerability threshold for schizophrenia. The second peak around menopause might be accounted for by the belated onsets of those women disposed to schizophrenia who until then were protected by estrogens.

Testing the Hypothesis in Animal Experiments

Together with Behrens, de Vry and Gattaz we were able to show in animal experiments that long-term estrogen treatment is capable of attenuating dopaminergic behaviour (Häfner et al. 1991a,b). The effects were clearly stronger in neonatal than in adult rats. We then looked for the underlying mechanism and found that estrogens significantly reduce D_2 receptor sensitivity in the brain. In the meantime our explicatory model, which is based on an effective neuromodulatory role of estrogens, has been supported by Sumner and Fink (1995) on an adjacent transmitter system. Using the same animal model, Sumner and Fink found that estradiol also significantly increases the number of serotonin receptors in the hippocampus and the frontal lobe. Woolley and McEwen (1994) found that the densities of dendritic spines and synapses on hippocampal CA1 pyramidal cells of the adult female rat also depend on ovarian steroid estradiol via a mechanism requiring activiation of *N*-methyl-D-aspartate (NMDA) receptors. Moreover, spine and synapse density fluctuate naturally as ovarian steroid levels vary across the estrous cycle. These mechanisms presumably add to the D_2 receptor-mediated neuromodulatory effect of estrogen.

We tested the applicability of our findings to humans together with Riecher-Rössler (Riecher-Rössler et al. 1994) in a controlled clinical study. A group of 32 women in acute episodes of schizophrenia and 29 controls in acute depressive episodes were compared for cyclical phases, plasma estrogen levels and symptom measures. Both the subjects and the controls had normal menstrual cycles. As shown in Table 7, all symptom measures except depressive symptomatology showed a significantly negative correlation [the Nurses' Observation Scale for Inpatient Evaluation (NOSIE) score has a reversed polarity] with the plasma estrogen level. In depressive controls no associations between symptom measures, plasma estrogen levels and menstrual phases were observed. This means that the same neuro-hormonal mechanism that we had traced in animal experiments is probably also active in human schizophrenia.

The mechanism that protects many schizophrenic women from developing the disorder until menopause is also involved in the only potent principle currently known in the treatment of schizophrenia, that is, the blockade of D_2 receptors by neuroleptics. In both cases psychotic symptoms are reduced and relapses or the onset of the disorder is delayed. But in neither case is the disorder cured. The similarity of the effects and the fact that the same principle is effective in both cases provides evidence for our estrogen hypothesis as an explanation of the sex difference in age of first onset.

It is very likely that the mechanism is not specific to schizophrenia. Indeed, dopamine blockade by neuroleptics is effective in a number of other excitative syndromes, too, such as mania, toxic or other exogenous psychoses. What we are presumably dealing with here is a transmitter system that involves D_2 and probably also NMDA receptors in the mesolimbic system, but which is as yet only poorly understood. Its functioning seems to be a precondition for the production of schizophrenic and other excitative syndromes. When the system is desensitized or blocked, the production of psychotic symptoms by the underlying disease process is at least impeded. In this way a considerable proportion of women disposed to schizophrenia is carried safely to menopause under the protective effect of estrogens.

Our findings provide evidence for the dopamine hypothesis of schizophrenia, which was temporarily discarded, but has cautiously been revived in recent years. The

Table 7. Means of individual correlation coefficients between estradiol curves and psychopathology ($n = 32$)

	Mean (SD)	p
BPRS, total score	−0.25 (0.41)	0.002
NOSIE, total score[a]	0.25 (0.49)	0.004
BFS, total score	−0.20 (0.43)	0.032
PDS, paranoid score	−0.17 (0.42)	0.029
PDS, depression score	−0.10 (0.52)	0.277 (NS)

SD, standard deviation; BPRS, Brief Psychiatric Rating Scale (Overall and Gorham 1962); NOSIE, Nurses' Observation Scale for Inpatient Evaluation (Honigfeld et a. 1976); BFS, Befindlichkeits-Skala; PDS, Paranoid-Depressivitäts-Skala (von Zerssen and Koeller 1976); NS, not significant.
[a]unlike the other scores, in the total NOSIE score a higher value means less psychopathology.
(From Riecher-Rössler et al. 1994)

evidence does quite definitely not involve the aetiology of the disorder. There is presumably a variety of causes that are capable of triggering the response pattern of schizophrenia as a "common final pathway". Besides developmental delays, cognitive deficits, exogenous psychoses, epileptic seizures, affective syndromes and dementia, schizophrenia is one of the very few final pathological patterns of response that the human brain has at its disposal, and it is not a single disease as Kraepelin had originally assumed.

References

Angermeyer MC, Kühn L (1988) Gender differences in age at onset of schizophrenia. Eur Arch Psychiatr Neurol Sci 237: 351–364

Biehl H, Maurer K, Schubart C, Krumm B, Jung E (1986) Prediction of outcome and utilization of medical services in a prospective study of first onset schizophrenics – results of a prospective 5-year follow-up study. Eur Arch Psychiatry Neurol Sci 236: 139–147

Choquet M, Ledoux S (1994) Epidémiologie et adolescence. In: Confrontations psychiatriques, vol 27, (no 35). Rhone-Poulenc rorer specia, Paris, pp 287–309

DiPaolo T, Falardeau P (1985) Modulation of brain and pituitary dopamine receptors by estrogens and prolactin. Prog Neuropsychopharmacol Biol Psychiatry 9: 473–480

Dohrenwend BP, Levav I, Shrout PE, Schwartz S, Naveh G, Link BG, Skodol AE, Stueve A (1992) Socioeconomic status and psychiatric disorders: the causation-selection issue. Science 255: 946–952

Fields JZ, Gordon JH (1982) Estrogen inhibits the dopaminergic supersensitivity induced by neuroleptics. Life Sci 30: 229–234

Häfner H, Riecher A, Maurer K, Löffler W, Munk-Jørgensen P (1989) How does gender influence age at first hospitalization for schizophrenia? A transnational case register study. Psychol Med 19: 903–918

Häfner H, Riecher A, Maurer K, Meissner S, Schmidtke A, Fätkenheuer B, Löffler W, an der Heiden W (1990) Ein Instrument zur retrospektiven Einschätzung des Erkrankungsbeginns bei Schizophrenie (instrument for the retrospective assessment of the onset of schizophrenia) – „IRAOS" – Entwicklung und Ergebnisse. Z Klin Psychol 19: 230–255

Häfner H, Behrens S, De Vry J, Gattaz WF (1991a) An animal model for the effects of estradiol on dopamine-mediated behavior: implications for sex differences in schizophrenia. Psychiatry Res 38: 125–134

Häfner H, Behrens S, de Vry J, Gattaz WF, Löffler W, Maurer K, Riecher-Rössler A (1991b) Warum erkranken Frauen später an Schizophrenie? Nervenheilkunde 10: 154–163

Häfner H, Riecher-Rössler A, Hambrecht M, Maurer K, Meissner S, Schmidtke A, Fätkenheuer B, Löffler W, an der Heiden W (1992) IRAOS: an instrument for the assessment of onset and early course of schizophrenia. Schizophr Res 6: 209–223

Häfner H, Maurer K, Löffler W, Bustamante S, an der Heiden W, Riecher-Rössler A, Nowotny B (1995) Onset and early course of schizophrenia. In: Häfner H, Gattaz WF (eds) Search for the causes of schizophrenia, vol. 3. Springer, Berlin Heidelberg New York (in press)

Hambrecht M, Maurer K, Sartorius N, Häfner H (1992) Transnational stability of gender differences in schizophrenia? An analysis based on the WHO study on determinants of outcome of severe mental disorders. Eur Arch Psychiatry Clin Neurosci 242: 6–12

Harrer S (1987) Über das Zusammenwirken von Östradiol und Dopamin bei der Verhaltenssteuerung von Säugern. Thesis, University of Stuttgart

Henn FA, McKinney WT (1987) Animal models in psychiatry. In: Meltzer HY (ed) Psychopharmacology: the third generation of progress. Raven, New York, pp 687–695

Jablensky A, Sartorius N, Ernberg G, Anker M, Korten A, Cooper JE, Day R, Bertelsen A (1992) Schizophrenia: manifestations, incidence and course in different cultures. A World Health Organization ten-country study. Psychol Med Monogr Suppl 20

Kraepelin E (1909–1915) Psychiatrie, 8th edn, vols 1–4. Barth, Leipzig

Lindelius R (1970) A study of schizophrenia. Acta Psychiatr Scand Suppl 216

Riecher-Rössler A, Häfner H, Stumbaum M, Maurer K, Schmidt R (1994) Can estradiol modulate schizophrenic symptomatology? Schizophr Bull 20: 203–214

Salokangas RKR, Stengard E, Räkköläinen v, Kaljonen IHA (1987) New schizophrenic patients and their families (English summary). Psychiatr Fenn 78: 119–216
Shepherd M, Watt D, Falloon I, Smeeton N (1989) The natural history of schizophrenia: a five-year follow-up study of outcome and prediction in a representative sample of schizophrenics. Psychol Med Monogr Suppl 15
Strömgren E (1935) Zum Ersatz des Weinbergschen „abgekürzten Verfahrens". Zugleich ein Beitrag zur Frage von der Erheblichkeit des Erkrankungsalters bei der Schizophrenie. Zeitschr Gesamte Neurol Psychiatr 153: 784–797
Sumner BEH, Fink G (1995) Oestradiol-17β in its positive feedback mode significantly increases 5-HT_{2a} receptor density in the frontal, cingulate and piriform cortex of the female rat. J Physiol (Lond) 483: 52
Tsuang MT, Fleming JA (1987) Long-term outcome of schizophrenia and other psychoses. In: Häfner H, Gattaz WF, Janzarik W (eds) Search for the causes of schizophrenia. Springer, Berlin Heidelberg New York pp 88–97
Woolley CS, McEwen BS (1994) Estradiol regulates hippocampal dendritic spine density via an N-Methyl-D-aspartate receptor-dependent mechanism. J Neurosci 14: 7680–7687

The Course of Psychiatric Disorders as a Diagnostic Tool

J. Angst

Why Classify By Course Characteristics?

Characteristics of the course of a disorder are of general prognostic value in terms of medical evaluation. Our knowledge of the statistical course of a disorder together with the individual previous history helps in predicting the future course and response to treatment. Psychiatry still lacks a classification based on pathogenesis, and for this reason, course is still used as a diagnostic criterion.

Elements of Course Used for Classification

The course of a disorder is a very complex phenomenon and different aspects are used to make a classification. Some major aspects are listed in Table 1.

The first is the *longitudinal change* or the stability of psychopathological syndromes, common examples of which are listed in Table 2. The most relevant point

Table 1. Elements of course suitable for classification

Longitudinal change of psychopathological syndromes
Severity and length
Frequency of episodes
Acuteness of onset
Development trends
Outcome: quality and degree of remission

Table 2. Longitudinal change or stability of psychopathological syndromes

Examples:	Depression → Schizoaffective Disorder → Schizophrenie residuum
	Depression → Mania → Bipolar disorder
	Depression → Panic → Agoraphobia
	Negative symptoms → Schizophrenia → Negative symptoms
	Migraine → Depression
	Anxiety disorders → Substance abuse
	Behavioral inhibition → Social Phobia → Alcoholism
Problems:	Comorbidity
	Primary-secondary distinction

is the comorbidity, in conjunction with the primary and secondary distinction based on the temporal sequence.

The *severity and length of manifestations* has been widely used in more recent diagnostic classification systems, examples of which are presented in Table 3. The subgroups obtained through this procedure may, however, seem to be highly artificial and reflect syndromes, rather than disorders, with similar psychopathology and similar genetic predispositions on a spectrum. The syndrome may, however, show different responses to treatments.

Table 3. Severity and length of manifestations

	Severity	Length
Minor depression	low	long
Brief depression	high	short
Major depression	high	long
Dysthymia	low	long
Chronic depression	high	long

A third factor is the *frequency of episodes*, which is important for the characterisation of affective or mood disorders and is also instrumental in making decisions about long-term medication (Table 4). Recurrent brief depression, recurrent brief hypomania, recurrent brief anxiety states, recurrent brief insomnia and 48 h-cycling in bipolar disorder are all examples of rapid or continuous cycling disorders.

Table 4. Frequency of episodes

Monophasic
Oligophasic
Polyphasic
Rapid cycling
Continuous cycling

A fourth aspect is the *acuteness of onset* of a disorder. This factor is closely linked with the length of psychopathological manifestations, which can be used in part to predict response to treatment.

A fifth aspect to be considered is the *longitudinal developmental trend* of course. Seasonality was, for instance, applied to the definition of seasonal affective disorder (SAD) (Table 5). It is well known that psychopathological manifestations change

Table 5. Development trend

Seasonal patterns
Increases or decreases in severity over recurrent episodes can be classified as:
Better
Continuous fluctuating
Worse

drastically over time in their severity and can shift between diagnostic thresholds, thus resulting in the distinctions between threshold and subthreshold psychiatric syndromes. Longitudinal development can be classified as: worse, continuous fluctuating, better. This classification was recently developed by Singer and Merikangas in the Zürich study.

Finally, *outcome* should be mentioned as an important element, defined by both quality and degree of remission (Table 6). This criterion formed a part of the classical nosology developed in the last century and has helped to distinguish mood disorders from schizophrenias.

Table 6. Outcome: quality and degree of remission

Full remission:	Symptom-free
Partial remission:	Residual symptoms, "dementia"
No remission = chronic:	Active process?
Suicide	

The rest of this chapter will focus on two issues of current controversy: (1) the "course" of a disorder as a criterion for affective and schizoaffective disorders and (2) "course" as a criterion for agoraphobia with panic (ICD) or panic with agoraphobia (DSM). Both of these issues have aroused controversy and called into question the correctness of the diagnostic classifications provided by the DSM-IV and ICD-10 today.

Affective and Schizoaffective Disorders

As illustrated in Fig. 1, schizoaffective disorders, defined as mood disorders with mood-incongruent psychotic features, are classified together in the DSM with mood disorders, whereas in the ICD-10, they form a third independent group somewhere between mood disorders and schizophrenias.

This classification has surfaced as a consequence of course characteristics and has its roots in the tradition of French psychopathology of the nineteenth century (Fig. 2). Esquirol (1838) and Baillarger (1853/54) described the longitudinal sequence of syndromal manic and depressive episodes, but it was Falret (1851) who recognised that manic and depressive manifestations belong to one and the same disorder (Pichot 1995).

In Germany, Kahlbaum (1863) was a pioneer in studying the course of psychiatric disorders. His friend and student Hecker (1871) expressed their approach most clearly as follows:

It is necessary

"when observing a patient to bear in mind the whole course of affective disorders. We shouldn't adopt an a priori principle of classification as a guideline and we shouldn't base [a classification] only on the presence or absence of a single symptom.

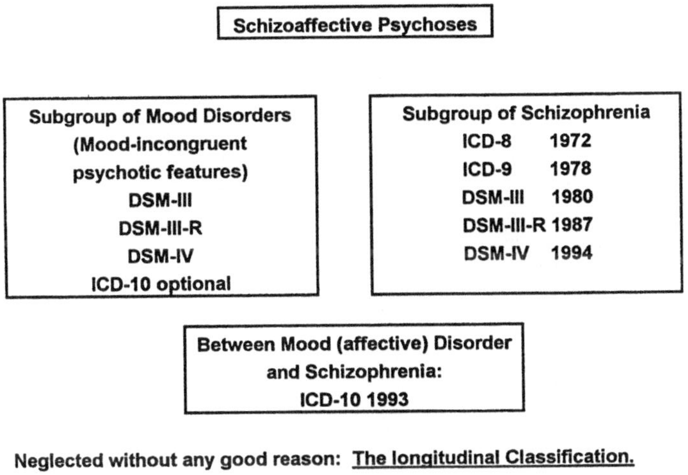

Fig. 1. Schizoaffective Psychoses in the DSM and ICD

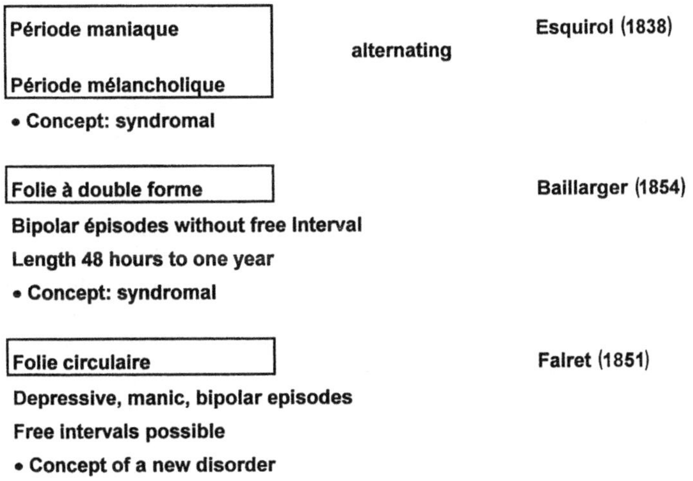

Fig. 2. Early history of bipolar disorder in French psychiatry

On the contrary, we should take all of the symptoms into equal consideration in our unibased observation, including the psychological and somatic elements and all of the remaining factors, in particular the etiology. Only in this way can psychiatry come closer to its aims of establishing types of diseases on a pathological-anatomical basis" (Schmidt-Degenhard 1983).

Kahlbaum (1874, 1882) was the first to base his complicated nosology on the outcome of psychiatric disorders. He distinguished clearly between two large groups of psychoses (Fig. 3). The first was "cyclothymia" or cyclic insanity, which consisted of mania, melancholia, hyperthymia and dysthymia and could never lead to

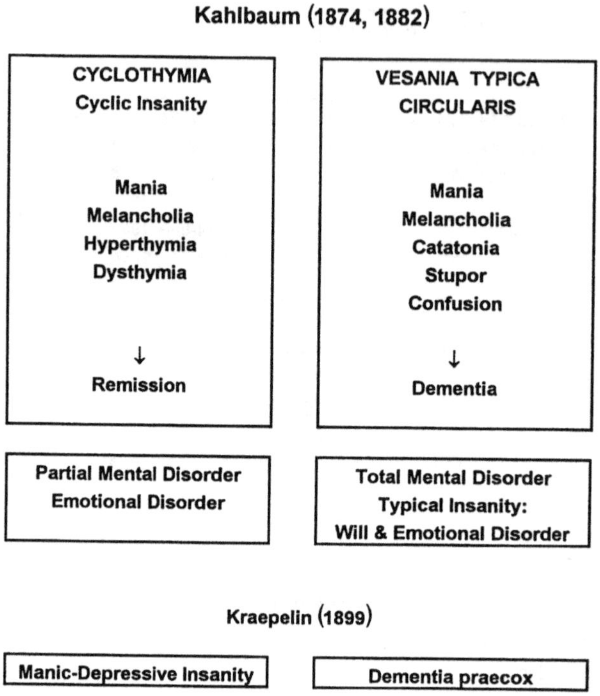

Fig. 3. From Kahlbaum to Kraepelin

dementia. These were recognised as being emotional disorders and, Kahlbaum thought, only partially affected the mind. In contrast to this first group, the second, which was termed "vesania typica circularis", could lead to dementia. Mania and melancholia were listed again in this group, along with catatonia, hebephrenia, stupor and confusions. This second group manifested, in his view, typical insanity as a complete mental disorder that affected the whole human mind. A dilemma was already inherent in his classification, with mania and melancholia designated as belonging to two classes of mental disorders with very different outcomes.

Kahlbaum's dichotomy was elaborated further by Kraepelin (1899) with much greater lucidity, when he included paranoid states in the concept of dementia praecox or schizophrenia, which leads ultimately to dementia. In both Kraepelin's (1899) and Bleuler's (1911) view, mania and melancholia could still occur within dementia praecox and schizophrenia. Today, this subgroup is labelled "schizoaffective disorders" and its nosological position is decidedly controversial, as shown by its classification under affective and schizoaffective disorders by the DSM or ICD.

An alternative view is the unitarian one, which considers schizoaffective disorders as forming a transitional group somewhere between affective and schizophrenic disorders on the broad spectrum of mental disorders. Schizoaffective disorders can include catatonic episodes, as described by Lange (1922), and they have a poorer prognosis than pure mood disorders. One interpretation, clearly adopted by the DSM, is to consider this subgroup of schizoaffectives to be a more severly affected group of mood disorders. This view certainly has some pragmatic value, for it has been proven that both affective and schizoaffective disorders require long-term phrophylactic medication with the same drugs. On the other hand, when judged from the genetic point of view, research has suggested that schizoaffective disorders, may share the genes for affective as well as for schizophrenic disorders, thus pointing to the intermediate position of this group (Angst 1966; Angst and Scharfetter 1979; Maier et al. 1992). It is probably wrong to merely subsume schizoaffective disorders under schizophrenia, as was done in ICD-9. In ICD-10, schizoaffective disorders received the status of a third indepedent group for the first time, which is a promising step forward.

Agoraphobia and Panic

The classification of agoraphobia and panic disorder is another issue surrounded by much controversy. Figure 4 illustrates the divergence between the classification of these conditions in the DSM-IV and the ICD-10. Two well-known experts in this field, Isaac Marks (1983, 1987, 1988) and Donald F. Klein (1983), continue to disagree profoundly on their classification.

Figure 4 illustrates clearly that the DSM gives precedence to panic disorder over phobias, whereas the ICD gives procedences to phobic disorders over panic. In an important paper by Marks (1988), it is stated that the classification of anxiety disorders by the presence of panic is "unsatisfactory", because panic is usually secondary to phobia and depression. Panic is not nearly as distinct a symptom as the DSM-III would have us believe (Tyrer 1986). Another paper published by Marks' group under the guidance of Basoglu et al. (1994) states that the relationship between

DSM Anxiety Disorders	ICD Anxiety Disorders
Panic Disorders	Phobic Anxiety Disorders
Panic Disorders + Agoraphobia	Agoraphobia with Panic
Agoraphobia	Agoraphobia
Social Phobia	Social Phobia
Specific Phobia	Specific Phobia
Generalized Anxiety Disorder	Other Anxiety Disorders
etc.	Panic Disorders
	Generalized Anxiety Disorders
	Mixed Anxiety and Depressive Disorders
	etc.

Fig. 4. Panic and agoraphobia in DSM and ICD

panic and avoidance is more complex than one of simple secondary conditioning. This point is crucial, as treatment results do not support the common emphasis on panic as a measure of treatment outcome in panic disorder with agoraphobia. The paper goes on to show that panic is often preceded by high levels of tonic anxiety. Epidemiological studies have clearly demonstrated that the majority of subjects with agoraphobia do not experience panic and just a minority of panic subjects experience agoraphobia. The relationship between the two is therefore of enduring interest.

The Zurich cohort study examined young subjects five times between the ages of 20 and 35. It collected data on age of first treatment and age of first onset and tried to trace, prospectively, the sequence of panic and agoraphobia. In Table 7 the age of first treatment of panic, anxiety, phobia and depression is listed for 11 cases meeting DSM-III criteria for panic disorder and DSM-III-R criteria for agoraphobia. In about half of all cases, panic developed simultaneously with phobia or depression or the latter were treated, at least, at a later date. A second group of subjects was treated first either for anxiety, phobia or depression and subsequently for panic disorder.

Table 8 shows the median of the age of first treatment for cases with both panic and agoraphobia versus panic alone or agoraphobia alone and illustrates the earlier treatment for anxiety, phobia and depression.

Our study also enabled subjects to date, in retrospect, the age of onset during different sections of the interview (Table 9). Panic, anxiety states, all phobias and depression were analysed. It is obvious that in the same subjects, phobias first occur

Table 7. Age of first treatment of DSM-III panic disorder with agoraphobia: 11 cases

Panic	Anxiety	Phobia	Depression
28	28	28	28
20	24	25	20
29	29	29	21
27	27	27	30
19	19	21	17
33	-	-	23
35	21	23	21
35	21	21	17
35	32	23	32
22	19	22	20
27	21	27	23

Table 8. Median age of first treatment for panic and/or agoraphobia

	DSM-III Diagnoses					
	Pan and Agos		Panic		Agoraphobia	
Treatment	*n*	M	*n*	M	*n*	M
Panic	11	26	31	28.5	18	-
Anxiety	11	21	32	21	45	23
Phobia	11	21	28	21	50	21
Depression	11	21	32	21	49	21

Pan, panic; Ago, agoraphobia; M, median.

Table 9. Median age of onset of panic and/or agoraphobia

	DSM-III Diagnoses					
	Pan and Ago (11)		Panic (32)		Agoraphobia (50)	
	n	M	*n*	M	*n*	M
Panic	11	21	31	21		-
Anxiety states	11	14	32	15.5	45	14
Phobias (all)	11	10		-	50	8.5
Depression	11	14	32	14.5	49	16

Fig. 5. Developmental sequence assessed in retrospect by age of onset

PHOBIA → ANXIETY/DEPRESSION → PANIC

in childhood, depression and anxiety states in adolescence and panic in early adulthood. We were therefore able to hypothesise in retrospect the developmental sequence from phobia to anxiety/depression and to panic, as shown in Fig. 5.

On the basis of the five interviews, we were also able to reconstruct the putative sequence of panic disorders and agoraphobia. The data are presented in Table 10. The association between the two syndromes was 3.4 higher than that expected by chance. We found an equal proportion of subjects (13%) showing a development from panic to secondary agoraphobia and from agoraphobia to secondary panic disorder. This finding corroborates with findings of Marks but conflicts with both DSM-III and DSM-IV concepts and, further, shows that combined cases of panic and agoraphobia can be subclassified into two subgroups. Whether this makes sense from the point of view of treatment is doubtful, according to the British findings reported by Basoglu, Marks et al. (1994).

Table 10. Temporal sequence of panic and agoraphobia in prospective data

DSM-III Panic → Agoraphobia 5/39 = 13%
Agoraphobia → DSM-III Panic 4/31 = 13%
Odds ratio = 3.4 (1.6–7.2)

The Zurich data also show clearly that panic attacks do not occur simply out of the blue but develop as a consequence of threshold or subthreshold anxiety states and/or depression. Anxiety states and depression usually develop about 6–7 years before panic disorder. We did not come across any subjects exhibiting panic disorder without such a previous history.

Lelliott et al. (1989), who investigated 57 patients with panic disorder and agoraphobia, found prodromal depression or anxiety in 52% of cases, prior to the first manifestation of panic. Agoraphobic avoidance preceded panic in 23% of cases. Spontaneous panic without a previous history of phobia, anxiety or depression may be rare in prospective investigations.

Conclusions

These two examples of agoraphobia/panic and schizoaffective disorders illustrate the importance of longitudinal studies. One should not just base such studies on defined patient samples; rather, prospective studies should also be conducted on subjects at risk or normal subjects, and the temporal sequence of psychopathological syndromes should be recorded carefully. With this broader emphasis, we are reminded of Kahlbaum's and Hecker's initial statement about the importance of studies concentrating on the course of a disorder.

References

Angst J (1966) Zur Ätiologie und Nosologie endogener depressiver Psychosen. Springer, Berlin Heidelberg New York

Angst J, Scharfetter C (1979) Subtypes of schizophrenia and affective disorders from a genetic viewpoint. In: Obiols J, Ballus C, Gonzales Monclus E, Pujol J (eds) Biological psychiatry today. Proceedings of the 2nd World Congress on Biological Psychiatry, Barcelona, Spain, 1978. Elsevier/North-Holland, Amsterdam, pp 351–357 (Developments in psychiatry, vol 2A)

Baillarger J (1853/54) Note sur un genre de folie dont les accès sont caractérisés par deux périodes régulières, l'une d dépression et l'autre d'excitation. Bull Acad Imp Med 19: 340–352

Baillarger J (1854) De la folie à double forme. Leçons faites à La Salpétrière dans le semestre d'été de 1854. Ann Med Psychol (Paris) 6: 369–391

Basoglu M, Marks IM, Kilic C, Swinson RP, Noshirvani H, Kuch K, O'Sullivan G (1994) Relationship of panic, anticipatory anxiety, agoraphobia and global improvement in panic disorder with agoraphobia treated with alprazolam exposure. Br J Psychiatry 164: 647–651

Bleuler E (1911) Dementia praecox oder Gruppe der Schizophrenien. In: Aschaffenburg G (ed) Handbuch der Psychiatrie, Spezieller Teil 4. Deuticke, Leipzig

Esquirol E (1838) Des maladies mentales considérées sous les rapports médical, hygiénique et médico-légal. Baillière, Paris

Falret JP (1851) De la folie circulaire ou forme de maladie mentale caractérisée par l'alternative régulière de la manie et de la mélancholie. Bull Acad Med (Paris)

Hecker E (1871) Die Hebephrenie. Ein Beitrag zur klinischen Psychiatrie. Virchows Arch Pathol Anat Physiol Klin Med 52: 203–218

Kahlbaum K (1863) Die Gruppirung der psychischen Krankheiten und die Eintheilung der Seelenstörungen. Kafemann, Danzig

Kahlbaum K (1874) Die Katatonie oder das Spannungsirresein. Eine klinische Form psychischer Krankheit. Hirschwald, Berlin

Kahlbaum K (1882) Über cyclisches Irresein (Vortrag). Correspondenzblatt des Verbandes der schlesischen Ärztevereine Irrenfreund 10

Klein DF (1983) Panic attacks in phobia treatment studies (in reply). Arch Gen Psychiatry 40: 1150

Kraepelin E (1899) Psychiatrie, 6th edn. Barth, Leipzig

Lange J (1922) Katatonische Erscheinungen im Rahmen manischer Erkrankungen. Springer, Berlin

Lelliott P, Marks I, McNamee G, Tobena A (1989) Onset of panic disorder with agoraphobia. Toward an integrated model. Arch Gen Psychiatry 46: 1000–1004

Maier W, Lichtermann D, Minges J, Heun R, Hallmayer J, Benkert O (1992) Schizoaffective disorder and affective disorder with mood-incongruent psychotic features: keep separate or combine? Evidence from a family study. Am J Psychiatry 149: 1666–1673

Marks I (1983) Panic attacks in phobia treatment studies (in reply). Arch Gen Psychiatry 40: 1150

Marks I (1987) Agoraphobia, panic disorder and related conditions in the DSM-IIIR and ICD-10. J Psychopharmacol 1: 6–12

Marks I (1988) The syndromes of anxious avoidance: classification of phobic and obsessive-compulsive phenomena. In: Noyes R Jr, Roth M, Burrows GD (eds) Classification, etiological factors and associated disturbances. Elsevier, Amsterdam (Handbook of anxiety, vol 2)

Pichot P (1995) The birth of the bipolar disorder. Eur Psychiatry 10: 1–10
Schmidt-Depenhard M (1983) Melancholie und Depression. Kohlhammer, Stuttgart, p 61
Singer, Merikangas (not yet published, personal communication)
Tyrer P (1986) Classification of anxiety disorders: a critique of DSM-III. J Affective Disord 11: 99–104

A Psychoanalytic Model for the Classification of Personality Disorders

O. F. KERNBERG

Categorical Versus Dimensional Models of Personality Disorders

A major problem regarding the classification of personality disorders is the understanding of the psychopathology of these disorders, that is, how the behavioral characteristics of any particular personality disorder relate to each other and to their particular predisposing and causative factors. Here, empirical researchers studying particular personality disorders (such as the borderline personality disorder, the narcissistic personality disorder, or the antisocial personality disorder) have attempted to pinpoint their etiological factors, but have found, again and again, that multiple factors appear to combine in the background of any particular personality disorder, without a clear answer as to how these factors relate to each other in codetermining a specific type of psychopathology (Marziali 1992; Paris 1994; Steinberg et al. 1994; Stone 1993a,b). Researchers proceeding with a dimensional model of classification usually carry out complex factor analyses of a great number of behavioral traits, leading to specific factors or a few overriding behavioral characteristics that, in different combinations, would seem to characterize the particular personality disorders described by clinicians (Benjamin 1992, 1993; Costa and Widiger 1994; Widiger and Frances 1994; Widiger et al. 1994). This approach links particular behaviors and lends itself to establishing a general theory that, in turn, integrates the major dimensions arrived at by statistical analyses. These dimensions, however, tend to have rather general relations to any particular personality disorder and, so far, seem to have been of little use for clinical purposes. [One notable exception may prove to be Lorna Smith Benjamin's (1992, 1993) "structural analysis of social behavior (SASB)" a model strongly influenced by contemporary psychoanalytic thinking.]

A currently dominant dimensional model, the five-factor model, has synthesized numerous factor analyses into the proposal that neuroticism, extroversion, openness, agreeableness, and conscientiousness constitute basic factors that may describe all "officially" accepted personality disorders in DSM-IV (Costa and Widiger 1994; Widiger et al. 1994). The problem, I believe, is whether these are really fundamental determinants of the organization of the normal personality or even of the personality disorders. An "equalization" of these character traits seems strange when applied to the subtleties of the clinical features of specific personality constellations. To develop factorial profiles for each personality disorder on the basis of those five factors has an eerie quality of unreality for the experienced clinician.

Those researchers who are inclined to maintain a categorical approach to the classification of personality disorders, usually clinical psychiatrists motivated to find specific disease entities, tend to proceed differently. They study the clinically prevalent combinations of pathological personality traits, carry out empirical research regarding the validity and reliability of clinical diagnoses, attempt to achieve a clear differentiation between personality disorders, and, of course, keep in mind the clinical relevance of their approaches (Akhtar 1992; Stone 1993a). This approach, pursued in DSM-III and DSM-IV, has helped to clarify – or at least to permit the clinical psychiatrist to become better acquainted with – some frequently seen personality disorders. The approach has been plagued, however, by the high degree of co-morbidity of the severe types of personality disorders, and by the unfortunate politicalization of decisionmaking, via committee, of what personality disorders to include and exclude in the official DSM system, and under what labels (Jonas and Pope 1992; Kernberg 1992; Oldham 1994). For this reason, a common personality disorder such as the hysterical personality disorder has remained excluded, while the depressive-masochistic personality disorder, excluded under DSM-III, has now reemerged under the heading "depressive personality disorder" in the appendix of DSM-IV, but shorn of its masochistic component (previously "tolerated" in DSM-III-R under the then still politically correct title of "self-defeating" personality disorder) (Kernberg 1992).

A major problem of both categorical and dimensional classification systems, in my view, has been the tendency to anchor the empirical research too closely to surface behavior, behavior that may serve very different functions according to the underlying personality structures. Thus, for example, what is seen as social timidity, social phobia, or inhibition, and may contribute to a diagnosis of either a schizoid or an avoidant personality may in fact reflect the cautiousness of a deeply paranoid individual, or the fear of exposure of a narcissistically grandiose individual, or a reaction formation against exhibitionistic tendencies in a hysterical individual. A related problem is the necessary dependency, in large-scale research efforts, on standardized inquiries or queationnaires that tend to be responded to, in part, according to the social values of particular personality traits: for example, to be excessively conscientious is more desirable than being irresponsible, to be generous is more valuable than being envious, etc. Our very diagnostic instruments need much further elaboration and may even have contributed to some of our problems.

It is far from my intention to suggest that a psychoanalytic exploration will resolve all existing problems. I cannot, at this point, present a satisfactory psychoanalytic model of classification of personality disorders. A psychoanalytic study of patients with personality disorders undergoing psychoanalytic treatment, however, facilitates the study of (a) the interrelationships among the patient's pathological personality traits, and of the relationships (b) between surface behavior and underlying psychological structure, (c) between various constellations of pathological behavior patterns as they change in the course of treatment, and (d) between motivation of behavior and psychological structure; it also allows (e) changes in the patient's behavior in response to shifts in dominant transference patterns to be examined.

Temperament, Character, and the Structure of the Normal Personality

I shall now present an updated view of my proposed psychoanalytic model for the classification of personality disorders, a model that incorporates significant contributions from other psychoanalytic researchers and theoreticians such as Rainer Krause (Krause 1988; Krause and Lutolf 1988), Vamik Volkan (1976, 1987), Michael Stone (1980, 1990, 1993a), and Salman Akhtar (1989, 1992). To begin, I shall refer to temperament and character as crucial aspects of personality. Temperament refers to the constitutionally given and largely genetically determined, inborn disposition to particular reactions to environmental stimuli, particularly to the intensity, rhythm, and thresholds of affective responses. I consider affective responses, particularly under conditions of peak affect states, the crucial determinants of the organization of the personality. Inborn differences in the activation of both positive, pleasurable, rewarding, and negative, painful, aggressive affects represent, I believe, the most important bridge between biological and psychological determinants of the personality (Kernberg 1994).

Cloninger et al. (1993) related particular neurochemical systems to temperamental dispositions he called "novelty seeking," "harm avoidance," "reward dependence," and "persistence", offering one such avenue relating biological systems to temperamental disposition. I should add, however, that I question Cloninger's direct translations of such dispositions into the specific types of personality disorders of the DSM classification system. Torgersen (1985, 1994), on the basis of his twin studies of genetic and environmental influences on the development of personality disorders, found that genetic influences appear significant only for the schizotypal personality disorder, and, for practical purposes, are significantly related to normal personality characteristics, but have very little relationship with specific personality disorders. Temperament alao includea inborn dispositions to cognitive organization and to motor behavior, such as the hormonal, particularly testosterone-derived, differences in cognitive functions and aspects of gender role identity that differentiate male and female behavior patterns. From the viewpoint of personality disorders, however, the affective aspects of temperament appear of fundamental importance.

In addition to temperament, character is another major component of personality. From a psychoanalytic perspective, I propose that character refers to the behavioral manifestations of ego identity, while the integration of the "self"concept and the integration of the concept of "significant others" are the intrapsychic structures that determine the dynamic organization of character. Character also includes all the behavioral aspects of what, in psychoanalytic terminology, is called "ego functions" and "ego structures." I see the personality as codetermined by temperament and character, and also by an additional intrapsychological structure, the superego. The moral and ethical dimension of the personality – from a psychoanalytic viewpoint, the integration of various layers of the superego – are an important component of the total personality. Personality itself, then, may be considered the dynamic integration of all behavior patterns derived from temperament, character, and internalized value systems (Kernberg 1976, 1980).

The normal personality ia characterized, first of all, by an integrated concept of the self and an integrated concept of significant others. These structural characteristics, jointly called "ego identity," (Erikson 1956; Jacobson, 1964) are reflected in an internal sense and an external appearance of self-coherence, and are a fundamental precondition for normal self-esteem, self-enjoyment, and zest for life. An integrated view of one's self assures the capacity for a realization of one's desires, capacities, and long-range commitments. An integrated view of significant others guarantees the capacity for an appropriate evaluation of others, empathy, and an emotional investment in others that implies a capacity for mature dependency while maintaining a consistent sense of autonomy as well.

A second structural characteristic of the normal personality, largely derived from and an expression of ego identity, is the presence of ego strength, particularly reflected in a broad spectrum of affect dispositions, capacity for affect and impulse control, and the capacity for sublimation in work and values (also contributed to importantly by the superego). Consistency, persistence, and creativity in work as well as in interpersonal relations are also largely derived from normal ego identity, as are the capacity for trust, reciprocity, and commitment to others, also importantly codetermined by superego functions (Kernberg 1975).

A third aspect of the normal personality is an integrated and mature superego, representing an internalization of value systems that is stable, depersonified, abstract, and individualized, and not excessively dependent on unconscious infantile prohibitions. Such a superego structure is reflected in a sense of personal responsibility; a capacity for realistic self-criticism; integrity as well as flexibility in dealing with the ethical aspecta of decisionmaking; a commitment to standards, values, and ideals; and the contribution to such a forementioned ego functions as reciprocity, trust, and investment in depth (Jacobson 1964).

A fourth aspect of the normal personality is an appropriate and satisfactory management of libidinal and aggressive impulses. It involves the capacity for a full expression of sensual and sexual needs integrated with tenderness and emotional commitment to a loved other, and a normal degree of idealization of the other and the relationship. Here, clearly, a freedom of sexual expression is integrated with ego identity and the ego ideal. In regard to aggression, a normal personality structure includes the capacity to sublimate in the form of self-assertion, to withstand attacks without excessive reaction, to react protectively, and to avoid turning aggression against the self. Again, ego and superego functions contribute to such an equilibrium.

The Motivational Aspects of Personality Organization: Affects and Drives

I have proposed in earlier work that the drives of libido and aggression are the hierarchically supraordinate integrations of corresponding pleasurable and rewarding, and painful and aversive affect states (Kernberg 1992, 1994). Affects are instinctive components of human behavior, that is, inborn dispositions common to all individuals of the human species. They emerge in the early stages of development and are gradually organized into drives as they are activated as part of early object relations. Gratifying, rewarding, pleasurable affects are integrated as libido as an overarching drive, and painful, aversive, negative affects are integrated as aggression as an overarching drive. Affects as inborn, constitutionally and genetically determined modes of reaction are triggered first by physiological and bodily experiences and then gradually in the context of the development of object relations.

Rage represents the core affect of aggression as a drive, and the vicissitudes of rage explain, in my view, the origins of hatred and envy – the dominant affects of severe personality disorders – as well as of normal anger and irritability. Similarly, the affect of sexual excitement constitutes the core affect of libido. Sexual excitement slowly and gradually crystallizes out of the primitive affect of elation and the early sensual responses to intimate bodily contact.

Krause (1988) has proposed that affects constitute a phylogenetically recent biological system evolved in mammals to signal the infant animal's emergency needs to its mother, corresponding to a parallel inborn capacity of the mother to read and respond to the infant's affective signals, thus protecting the early development of the dependent infantile mammal. Affectively driven development of object relations – in other words, of real and fantasized interpersonal interactions that are internalized as a complex world of self and object representations in the context of affective interactions – I propose, constitute the determinants of unconscious mental life and of the structure of the psychological apparatus. Affects, in short, are the building blocks of the drives; they are also signals that the drives have been activated in the context of a particular internalized object relation. We can trace this process in the transference developments during psychoanalysis and psychoanalytic psychotherapy.

I believe this theory of motivation permits us to account for the concept of inborn dispositions to excessive or inadequate affect activation, thereby doing justice to the genetic and constitutional variations of intensity of drives reflected, for example, in the intensity, rhythm, and thresholds of affect activation commonly designated as temperament. This theory equally permits us to incorporate the effects of physical pain, psychological trauma, and severe disturbances in early object relations as contributing to intensifying aggression as a drive by triggering intense negative affects. In short, I believe, the theory does justice to Freud's (1915) statement that drives occupy an intermediate realm between the physical and the psychological realms.

Recent studies of alteration in neurotransmitter systems in severe personality disorders, particularly in the borderline personality disorder, although still tentative and open to varying interpretations, point to the possibility that neurotransmitters are related to specific distortions in affect activation (Stone 1993a,b). Abnormalities in the adrenergic and cholinergic systems, for example, may be related to general affective instability; deficits in the dopaminergic system may be related to a disposition toward transient psychotic symptoms in borderline patients; and impulsive, aggressive, self-destructive behavior may be facilitated by a lowered function of the serotonergic system (deVagvar et al. 1994; Steinberg et al. 1994; Stone 1993a,b; van Reekum et al. 1994; Yehuda et al. 1994). In general, genetic dispositions to temperamental variations in affect activation would seem to be mediated by alterations in neurotransmitter systems, providing a potential link between the biological determinants of affective response and the psychological triggers of specific affects.

These aspects of inborn dispositions to the activation of aggression mediated by the activation of aggressive affect states are complementary to the now well-established findings that structured aggressive behavior in infants may derive from early, severe, chronic physical pain, and that habitual aggressive teasing interactions with mothers are followed by similar behaviors in infants, as we know from the work of Galenson (1986) and Fraiberg (1983). Grossman's (1986, 1991) convincing arguments in favor of the direct transformation of chronic intense pain into aggression provides a theoretical context for the earlier observations of the battered-child syndrome. The impressive findings of the prevalence of physical and sexual abuse in the history of borderline patients confirmed by investigators both in the U.S. and abroad (Marziali 1992; Perry and Herman 1993; van der Kolk et al. 1994) provide additional evidence of the influence of trauma on the development of severe manifestations of aggression.

I am stressing the importance of this model for our understanding of the pathology of aggression because the exploration of severe personality disorders consistently finds the pathologic predominance of aggression as a major aspect of their psychopathology. One key dynamic of the normal personality is the dominance of libidinal strivings over aggressive ones. Drive neutralization, according to my formulation, implies the integration of libidinally and aggressively invested, originally split, idealized and persecutory internalized object relations, a process that leads from the state of separation-individuation to that of object constancy, and culminates in an integrated concept of the self, an integrated concept of significant others, and the integration of derivative affect states from the aggressive and libidinal series into the toned-down, discrete, elaborated, and complex affect disposition of the phase of object constancy.

While a central motivational aspect of severe personality disorders is the development of inordinate aggression and the related psychopathology of aggressive affect expression, the dominant pathology of the less severe personality disorders – which, in contrast to borderline personality organization (the severe personality disorders), I have called "neurotic personality organization" (Kernberg 1975, 1976, 1980, 1984) – is the pathology of libido, or of sexuality in an ordinary sense. This field includes particularly the hysterical, the obsessive-compulsive, and the depressive-masochistic personalities, although it is most evident in the hysterical personality disorder (Kernberg 1984). In contrast, sexuality is usually "coopted" by aggression in borderline personality organization, that is, sexual behavior and interaction are intimately condensed with aggressive aims, which severely limits or distorts sexual intimacy, love relations, and fosters the abnormal development of paraphilias with their heightened condensation of sexual and aggressive aims.

A Psychoanalytic Nosology

My own classification of personality disorders centers on the dimension of severity. Severity ranges from (a) psychotic personality organization, (b) borderline personality organization, to (c) neurotic personality organization. *Psychotic personality* organization is characterized by a lack of integration of the concept of self and significant others, that is, identity diffusion, a predominance of primitive defensive operations centering around splitting, and loss of reality testing. I only need to clarify here that a basic function of the defensive operations of splitting and its derivatives (projective identification, denial, primitive idealization, omnipotence, omnipotent control, and devaluation) is to maintain separate the idealized and persecutory internalized object relations derived from the early developmental phases predating object constancy: that is, the stage when aggressively determined internalizations strongly dominate the internal world of object relations, in order to prevent the overwhelming control or destruction of ideal object relations by aggressively infiltrated ones. This primitive constellation of defensive operations centering around splitting thus attempts to protect the capacity to depend on good objects and escape from terrifying aggression.

Reality testing refers to the capacity to differentiate self from nonself and intrapsychological from external stimuli, and to maintain empathy with ordinary social criteria of reality, all of which are typically lost in the psychoses, and manifested particularly in hallucinations and delusions (Kernberg 1976, 1984). The loss of reality testing reflects the lack of differentiation between self and object representations under conditions of peak affect states, that is, a structural persistence of the symbiotic stage of development, its pathological hypertrophy, so to speak. All patients with psychotic personality organization really represent atypical forms of psychosis. Therefore, strictly speaking, psychotic personality organization represents an exclusion criterion for the personality disorders in a clinical sense.

Borderline personality organization is also characterized by identity diffusion and the same predominance of primitive defensive operations centering on splitting, but is distinguished by the presence of good reality testing, reflecting the differentiation between self and object representations in the idealized and persecutory sector, characteristic of the separation-individuation phase (Kernberg 1975). Actually, this category includes all the severe personality disorders in clinical practice. Typical personality disorders included here are the borderline personality disorder in a DSM sense, the schizoid and schizotypal personality disorders, the paranoid personality disorder, the hypomanic personality disorder, hypochondriasis (a syndrome which has many characteristics of a personality disorder proper), the narcissistic personality disorder (including the syndrome of malignant narcissism), and the antisocial personality disorder.

All these patients present identity diffusion, the manifestations of primitive defensive operations, and many evince varying degrees of superego deterioration (antisocial behavior). A particular group of patients typically suffer from significant disorganization of the superego, namely, the narcissistic personality disorder, the syndrome of malignant narcissism, and the antisocial personality disorder.

All the personality disorders within the borderline spectrum present, because of the identity diffusion, severe distortions in their interpersonal relations – particularly problems in intimate relations with others, lack of consistent goals in terms of commitment to work or profession, uncertainty and lack of direction in their lives in many areas, and varying degrees of pathology in their sexual life. They often present an incapacity to integrate tenderness and sexual feelings, and they may show a chaotic sexual life with multiple polymorphously perverse infantile tendencies. The most severe cases, however, may present with a generalized inhibition of all sexual responses derived from a lack of sufficient activation of sensuous responses in the early relation with the caregiver, an overwhelming predominance of aggression that interferes with sensuality (rather than even coopting it for aggressive aims). All these patients also evince nonspecific manifestations of ego weakness, that is, lack of anxiety tolerance, of impulse control, and of sublimatory functioning in terms of an incapacity for consistency, persistence, and creativity in work.

An additional group of personality disorders also presents the characteristics of borderline personality organization, but these patients are able to maintain more satisfactory social adaptation, and are usually more effective in obtaining some degree of intimacy in object relations and in integrating sexual and tender impulses. Thus, in spite of presenting identity diffusion, they also evince sufficient non-conflictual development of some ego functions, superego integration, and a benign cycle of intimate involvements, capacity for dependency gratification, and a better adaptation to work that make for quantitatively significant differences. They constitute what might be called a "higher level" of borderline personality organization or an intermediate level of personality disorder. This group includes the cyclothymic personality, the sadomasochistic personality, the infantile or histrionic personality, and the dependent personalities, as well as some better functioning narcissistic personality disorders.

The next level of personality disorder, namely, *neurotic personality organization*, is characterized by normal ego identity and the related capacity for object relations in depth, ego strength reflected in anxiety tolerance, impulse control, sublimatory functioning, effectiveness and creativity in work, and a capacity for sexual love and emotional intimacy disrupted only by unconscious guilt feelings reflected in specific pathological patterns of interaction in relation to sexual intimacy. This group includes the hysterical personality, the depressive-masochistic personality, the obsessive personality, and many so-called avoidant personality disorders, in other words, the "phobic character" of psychoanalytic literature (which, in my view, remains a problematic entity).

Having thus classified personality disorders in terms of their severity, let us now examine particular continuities within this field that represent psychopathological links in this network, one might say, of related personality disorders. The borderline personality disorder and the schizoid personality disorder may be described as the simplest form of personality disorders, reflecting a fixation at the level of separation-individuation, with the "purest" expression of the general characteristics of borderline personality organization mentioned. Fairbairn (1954), in fact, described the schizoid personality as the prototype of all personality disorders, and provided an understanding of the psychodynamics of these patients unsurpassed to this day. He described the splitting operations separating "good" and "bad" internalized object relations the self and object representation dyads of the split-off object relations, the consequent impoverishment of interpersonal relations, and their replacement by a defensive hypertrophy of fantasy life. The borderline personality disorder in DSM terms presents similar dynamic characteristics, but with an expression of this pathology in impulsive interactions in the interpersonal field, in contrast to the expression of the pathology in the patient's fantasy life and social withdrawal in the schizoid personality (Akhtar 1992; Stone 1994).

The schizotypal personality reflects the most severe form of schizoid personality disorder, while the paranoid personality evinces an increase of aggression in comparison to the schizoid personality disorder, with a dominance of projective mechanisms and a defensive self-idealization related to the efforts to control an external world of persecutory figures. If splitting per se dominates in the borderline and schizoid personality disorders, projective identification dominates in the paranoid personality disorder. The hypochondriacal syndrome reflects a projection of persecutory objects onto the interior of the body: hypochondriacal personalities usually also show strong paranoid and schizoid characteristics.

The borderline personality proper presents an intensity of affect activation and lack of affect control which also suggests the presence of a temperamental factor; but the integration of aggressive and libidinal affects obtained in the course of treatment often brings about a remarkable toning down and modulation of affect response. The increase of impulse control and affect tolerance resulting during treatment illustrates that splitting mechanisms are central in that pathology (overcoming splitting, that is, integrating mutually split affects, leads to their integration, toning down, and maturation). The hypomanic personality disorder, in contrast, appears to include a pathology of affect activation that points to temperamental predisposition, which probably also holds true for its milder form, the cyclothymic personality.

Borderline personality disorders presenting intense aggression may evolve into the sadomasochistic personality disorder. If a disposition to strong sadomasochism becomes incorporated into or controlled by a relatively healthy superego structure (which also incorporates a depressive potential into a disposition to guilt-laden responses), and ego identity is achieved, the conditions for a depressive-masochistic personality disorder are also present. The depressive-masochistic personality may be considered the highest level of two developmental lines that go from the borderline personality through the sadomasochistic to the depressive-masochistic on the one hand, and from the hypomanic through the cyclothymic personality disorders to the depressive masochistic one, on the other. This entire area of personality disorders thus reflects the internalization of object relations under conditions of abnormal affective development or affect control.

When a severe inborn disposition to aggressive reactions, early trauma, severe pathology of early object relations, physical illness, and/or sexual and physical abuse intensify the dominance of aggression in the personality structure, a particular pathology of aggression may develop that includes, as we have already seen, the paranoid personality, hypochondriasis, and sadomasochism; it may also penetrate the field of the narcissistic personality disorder.

The narcissistic personality disorder is of particular interest because, in contrast to the clear indication of identity diffusion of all other personality disorders included in borderline personality organization, in the narcissistic personality a lack of integration of the concept of significant others goes hand in hand with an integrated, but pathological, grandiose self. This pathological grandiose self replaces the underlying lack of integration of a normal self (Akhtar 1989; Plakun 1989; Ronningstam and Gunderson 1989).

When intense pathology of aggression dominates in a narcissistic personality structure, the pathological grandiose self may become infiltrated by ego-syntonic aggression, with the development of a grandiosity combined with ruthlessneas, sadism, or hatred that translates into the syndrome of malignant narcissism, that is, a combination of narcissistic personality, antisocial behavior, ego-syntonic aggression, and paranoid tendencies. This syndrome, I have proposed, is intermediate between the narcissistic personality disorder and the antisocial personality disorder proper, in which a total absence or deterioration of superego functioning has occurred (Kernberg 1992). The antisocial personality disorder in a strict sense (Akhtar 1992; Bursten 1989; Hare 1986; Kernberg 1984) usually reveals, in psychoanalytic exploration, severe underlying paranoid trends, together with a total incapacity for any nonexploitive investment in significant others. The total absence of the capacity for guilt feelings, of any concern for self and others, the incapacity to identify with any moral or ethical value in self or others, and an incapacity to project a dimension of personal future characterize this personality disorder, thus differentiating it from the less severe syndrome of malignant narcissism, in which some commitment to others, and a capacity for authentic guilt feelings is still present. Prognostically, the extent to which nonexploitive object relations – the capacity for significant investment in others – is still present, and the extent to which antisocial behaviors dominate, are the most important indicators for any psychotherapeutic approach to the personality disorders (Kernberg 1975; Stone 1990).

At a higher level of development, the obsessive-compulsive personality may be conceived as one in which inordinate aggression has been neutralized by its absorption into a well-integrated but excessively sadistic superego, leading to perfectionism, self-doubts, and a chronic need to control the environment as well as the self characteristic of this personality disorder.

While the infantile or histrionic personality disorder is a milder form of the borderline personality disorder and still within the borderline spectrum, the hysterical personality disorder represents a higher-level type of the infantile or histrionic personality disorder, within the neurotic spectrum of personality organization. As I have described in earlier work (Kernberg 1992), in the hysterical personality the emotional lability, extroversion, and dependent and exhibitionistic traits of the histrionic personality are restricted to the sexual realm, while these patients are able to have normally deep, mature, committed, and differentiated object relations in other areas. In addition, in contrast to the sexual "freedom" of the typical infantile personality, the hysterical personality often presents a combination of pseudohypersexuality and sexual inhibition, with a particular differentiation of the relationships to men and women that contrasts with the nonspecific orientation of both genders of the infantile or histrionic personality.

Finally, the depressive-masochistic personality disorder (Kernberg 1992), the highest-level outcome of the pathology of depressive affect as well as that of sadomasochism characteristic of a dominance of aggression in primitive object relations, presents not only a well-integrated superego (as in all other personalities with neurotic personality organization), but an extremely punitive superego. This superego predisposes the patient to self-defeating behavior, reflects an unconscious need to suffer as an expiation for guilt feelings or a precondition for sexual pleasure, a reflection of the oedipal dynamics characterizing this high-level spectrum of personality disorders. The excessive dependency and easy frustration of dependency needs of these patients goes hand in hand with their "faulty metabolism" of aggression, where depression ensues when an aggressive response would have been appropriate, and an excessivly aggressive response to the frustration of their dependency needs may rapidly turn into a renewed depressive response as a

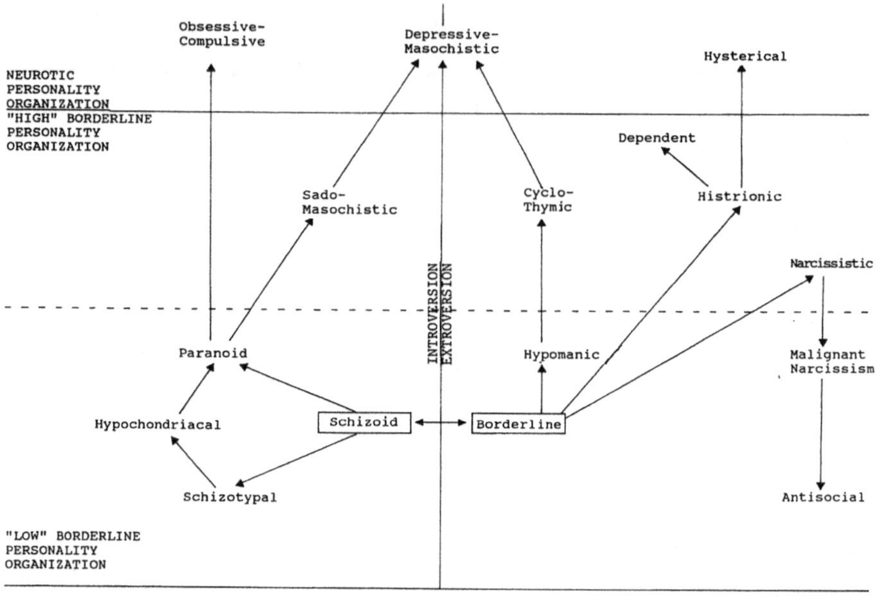

Fig. 1. Relationships among personality disorders and their classification into neurotic and borderline personality organization

consequence of excessive guilt feelings. Figure 1 summarizes the relationship among all the personality disorders mentioned, and represents their overall classification into neurotic and borderline personality organization.

References

Abraham K (1920) Manifestations of the female castration complex. In: Selected papers on psycho-analysis. Hogarth, London, pp 338–369

Abraham K (1921–1925) Psycho-analytical studies on character formation. In: Selected papers on psycho-analysis. Hogarth, London, pp 370–417

Akhtar S (1989) Narcissistic personality disorder: descriptive features and differential diagnosis. In: Kernberg OF (ed) Narcissistic personality disorder: psychiatric clinics of North America. Saunders, Philadelphia, pp 505–530

Akhtar S (1992) Broken structures. Aronson, Northvale

American Psychiatric Association (1968) Diagnostic and statistical manual of mental disorders: DSM-II. APA, Washington

American Psychiatric Association (1980) Diagnostic and statistical manual of mental disorders: DSM-III. APA, Washington

American Psychiatric Association (1994) Diagnostic and statistical manual of mental disorders: DSM-IV. APA, Washington

Benjamin LS (1992) An interpersonal approach to the diagnosis of borderline personality disorder. In: Clarkin JF et al. (eds) Borderline personality disorder. Guilford, New York, pp 161–198

Benjamin LD (1993) Interpersonal diagnosis and treatment of personality disorders. Guilford, New York

Bursten B (1989) The relationship between narcissistic and antisocial personalities. In: Kernberg

OF (ed) Narcissistic personality disorder: psychiatric clinics of North America. Saunders, Philadelphia, pp 571–584
Clarkin JF et al. (1992) Psychodynamic psychotherapy of the borderline patient. In: Clarkin JF et al. (eds) Borderline personality disorder. Guilford, New York, pp 268–287
Cloninger CR et al. (1993) A psychobiological model of temperament and character. Arch Gen Psychiatry 50: 975–990
Costa PT, Widiger TA (1994) Introduction. In: Costa PT, Widiger T (eds) Personality disorders and the five-factor model of personality. American Psychological Association, Washington, pp 1–10
DeVagvar ML et al. (1994) Impulsivity and serotonin in borderline personality disorder. In: Silk KR (ed) Biological and neurobehavioral studies of borderline personality disorder. American Psychiatric Press, Washington, pp 23–40
Erikson EH (1956) The problem of ego identity. 4: 56–121
Fairbairn W (1954) An object-relations theory of the personality. Basic, New York
Fenichel O (1945) The psychoanalytic theory of neurosis. Norton, New York
Fraiberg A (1983) Pathological defenses in infancy. Psychoanal 60: 612–635
Freud S (1980) Character and anal erotism. S.E. 9: 167–175
Freud S (1915) Instincts and their vicissitudes. S.E. 14: 109–140
Freud S (1931) Libidinal types. S.E. 21: 215–220
Galenson E (1986) Some thoughts about infant psychopathology and aggressive development. Inter Rev Psychoanal 13: 349–354
Grossmann W (1986) Notes on masochism: a discussion of the history and development of a psychoanalytic concept. I. Psychoanal Q 55: 379–413
Grossman W (1991) Pain, aggression, fantasy, and concepts of sadomasochism. Psychoanal Q 60: 22–52
Hare RD (1986) Twenty years of experience with the Cleckley psychopath. In: Reid WH et al. (eds) Unmasking the psychopath. Norton, New York, pp 3–27
Jacobson E (1964) The self and object world. International Universities Press, New York
Jonas JM, Pope HG (1992) Axis I comorbidity of borderline personality disorder: clinical implications. In: Clarkin JF et al. (eds) Borderline personality disorder. Guilford, New York, pp 149–160
Kernberg OF (1975) Borderline conditions and pathological narcissism. Aronson, New York
Kernberg OF (1976) Object relations theory and clinical psychoanalysis. Aronson, New York
Kernberg OF (1980) Internal world and external reality: object relations theory applied. Aronson, New York
Kernberg OF (1984) Severe personality disorders: psychotherapeutic strategies. Yale University Press, New Haven
Kernberg OF (1989) The narcissistic personality disorder and the differential diagnosis of antisocial behavior. In: Kernberg OF (ed) Narcissistic personality disorder: psychiatric clinics of North America. Saunders, Philadelphia, pp 553–570
Kernberg OF (1992) Aggression in personality disorder and perversions. Yale University Press, New Haven
Kernberg OF (1993) The psychotherapeutic treatment of borderline patients. In: Paris J (ed) Borderline personality disorder. American Psychiatric Press, Washington, pp 261–284
Kernberg OF (1994) Aggression, trauma, and hatred in the treatment of borderline patients. In: Share I (ed) Borderline personality disorder: the psychiatric clinics of North America. Isiah Share (ed) Saunders, Philadelphia, pp 701–714
Kernberg OF et al. (1989) Psychodynamic psychotherapy of borderline patients. Basic, New York
Klein M (1952) The origins of transference. In: Envy and gratitude. Basic, New York, pp 48–56
Krause R (1988) Eine Taxonomie der Affekte und ihre Anwendung auf das Verständnis der frühen Störungen. Psychother Med Psychol 38: 77–86
Krause R, Lutolf P (1988) Facial indicators of transference processes in psychoanalytical treatment. In: Dahl H, Kochele H (eds) Psychoanalytic process research strategies. Springer, Berlin Heidelberg New York, pp 257–272
Mahler M, Furer M (1968) On human symbiosis and the vicissitudes of individuation. International Universities Press, New York
Mahler M, Pine F, Bergman A (1975) The psychological birth of the human infant. Basic, New York
Marziali E (1992) The etiology of borderline personality disorder: developmental factors. In: Clarkin JF et al. (eds) Borderline personality disorder. Guilford, New York, pp 27–44
Oldham JM (1994) Personality disorders. JAMA 272: 1770–1776
Paris J (1994) Borderline personality disorder. American Psychiatric Press, Washington

Perry JC, Herman JL (1993) Trauma and defense in the etiology of borderline personality disorder. In: Paris J (ed) Borderline personality disorder. American Psychiatric Press, Washington, pp 123–140
Plakun E (1989) Narcissistic personality disorder: a validity study and comparison to borderline personality disorder. In: Kernberg OF (ed) Narcissistic personality disorder: psychiatric clinics of North America. Saunders, Philadelphia, pp 603–620
Ronningstam E, Gunderson J (1989) Descriptive studies on narcissistic personality disorder. In: Kernberg OF (ed) Narcissistic personality disorder: psychiatric clinics of North America. Saunders, Philadelphia, pp 585–602
Steinberg BJ et al. (1994) The cholinergic and noradrenergic neurotransmitter systems and affective instability in borderline personality disorder. In: Silk KR (ed) Biological and neurobehavioral studies of borderline personality disorder. American Psychiatric Press, Washington, pp 41–62
Stone M (1980) The borderline syndromes. McGraw-Hill, New York
Stone M (1990) The fate of borderline patients. Guilford, New York
Stone M (1993a) Abnormalities of personality. Norton, New York
Stone M (1993b) Etiology of borderline personality disorder: psychobiological factors contributing to an underlying irritability. In: Paris J (ed) Borderline personality disorder. American Psychiatric Press, Washington, pp 87–102
Stone M (1994) Characterologic subtypes of the borderline personality disorder: with a note on prognostic factors. In: Share I (ed) Borderline personality disorder: the psychiatric clinics of North America. Saunders, Philadelphia, pp 773–784
Torgersen AM (1985) Temperamental differences in infants and 6-year-old children: a follow-up study of twins. In: Stelan J, Farley FH, Gale H (eds) The biological basis of personality and behavior: theories, measurement, techniques, and development. Hemisphere, Washington
Torgersen AM (1994) Genetics of personality disorder. 1st European Congress on Disorders of Personality, June 16, Nijmegen
Van der Kolk BA et al. (1994) Trauma and the development of borderline personality disorder. In: Share I (ed) Borderline personality disorder: the psychiatric clinics of North America. Isiah Share (ed) Saunders, Philadelphia, pp 715–730
Van Reekum R et al. (1994) Impulsivity in borderline personality disorder. In: Silk KR (ed) Biological and neurobehavioral studies of borderline personality disorder. American Psychiatric Press, Washington, pp 1–22
Volkan V (1976) Primitive internalized object relations. New York: International Universities Press, New York
Volkan V (1987) Six steps in the treatment of borderline personality organization. Aronson, Northvale
Widiger TA, Frances AJ (1994) Toward a dimensional model for the personality disorders. In: Costa PT, Widiger T (eds) Personality disorders and the five-factor model of personality. American Psychological Association, Washington, pp 19–40
Widiger TA et al. (1994) A description of the DSM-III-R and DSM-IV personality disorders with the five-factor model of personality. In: Costa PT, Widiger T (eds) Personality disorders and the five-factor model of personality. American Psychological Association, Washington, pp 41–56
Yehuda R et al. (1994) Peripheral catecholamine alterations in borderline personality disorder. In: Silk KR (ed) Biological and neurobehavioral studies of borderline personality disorder. American Psychiatric Press, Washington, pp 63–90

Functional Psychopathology: An Essential Diagnostic Step in Biological Psychiatric Research

H. M. van Praag

Nosology: The Apple of Psychiatry's Eye

In experimental psychiatry, nosology has been and still is the prevailing diagnostic philosophy. Nosology presumes the existence of discrete psychiatric diseases, each with their own identity in terms of phenomenology, causation, prognosis and treatment outcome. "Nature, in the production of diseases, is uniform and consistent; so much so, that for the same disease in different persons the symptoms are for the most part the same; and the self-same phenomena that you could observe in the sickness of a Socrates you would observe in the sickness of a simpleton." Such was the terse way in which Sydenham, in 1682, formulated the nosological standpoint (Pichot 1994).

In other words, having cross-sectionally diagnosed a particular disorder, causation, course and outcome are thought to be in large measure predictable. Nosology is the central premise of biological psychiatric research. Its goal is to find "markers" and eventually causes of separate disease entities.

I have been a nosological skeptic all my professional life, because I was struck by the many observations that didn't fit and seemed to even be irreconcileable with the nosological adage (Van Praag 1992a).

Between patients considered to suffer from the same disease, the diversity in symptoms is often striking. The behavior of a hebephrenic patient, for instance, is profoundly different from one suffering from paranoid schizophrenia. Little of their psychopathology can be brought under the same denominator. Moreover, within one patient, the symptomatology is often far from constant. Not infrequently, over time, one has to switch diagnoses. Furthermore, a particular diagnosis made at a certain point in time predicts little in terms of treatment response and course. For instance, little additional information is gained by using neither Kraepelin's subdivision of schizophrenia or the subgroupings distinguished in the latest DSM editions, nor do they seem to have much bearing on such variables as genetic loading, premorbid personality structure and social disability (Tsuang et al. 1990; Wolkowitz et al. 1990; Lindenmayer et al. 1994; Strakowski 1994; Roy and Crowe 1994; Ram et al. 1992).

Even more disturbing to me was the observation that relatively few patients showed a particular disease in a complete and pure form. Many appeared to qualify for a variety of disorders or showed a patchwork of parts of different syndromes or disorders. Comorbidity – as this phenomenon is presently called – is, of course, not a new discovery. The program on the biology of depression, which we started in the late 1950s was from the beginning plagued by the fact that so many patients, with vital depression (the syndrome of endogenous depression), a syndrome we were particularly interested in and had defined operationally (Van Praag et al. 1965), showed the syndrome in an incomplete form and/or in conjunction with other disorders. The combination with (to use the nomenclature of the time) free floating anxiety (presently called generalized anxiety disorder) occurred in 65% of the patients, with hyperventilation syndrome (panic disorder) in 28% and obsessive compulsive neurosis (obsessive compulsive disorder) in 7%.

In short, it appeared that: (1) nosologically based diagnoses made it hard to characterize a particular patient in any detail; (2) the predictive validity of many diagnostic constructs is limited; and (3) comorbidity burdens experimental psychiatry with formidable problems. The last problem I considered to be the thorniest (Van Praag 1995c). How can one study the biology of a given disorder, its epidemiology, its course, and the results of biological and psychological therapeutic interventions, if more often than not the disorder appears hand in hand with several others? Which disorder are we actually studying?

Nosology and Biological Psychiatry

Biological psychiatry, typically, has felt the limitations of the nosological approach most dramatically. Thirty five years of intensive research efforts have yielded a vast amount of often interesting, biological data, little of which, however, has had any practical diagnostic significance. In diagnosing most psychiatric disorders biology plays a subordinate role at best. This could be due to shortcomings of the biological methodology or to flaws in the diagnostic process. I consider the latter explanation more plausible than the former.

Psychopharmacology provides another case in point. The classification of psychotropic drugs has been nosologically based, but over the years it has become apparent that this principle poorly fits the goal. Antidepressants are indeed effective in depression, but likewise in various anxiety disorders (Rickels et al. 1993; Den Boer and Sitsen 1994; Den Boe et al. 1994). Several anxiolytics, particulary the 5-hydroxytryptamine $(5\text{-HT})_{1A}$ agonists, can act as antidepressants as well (Pecknold 1994). The beneficial effect of neuroleptics is not restricted to schizophrenia but extends to all types of psychotic disorders. Lithium exerts a prophylactic effect in bipolar and unipolar depressions but in other cyclic disorders, such as schizoaffective disorders, as well (Jefferson and Greist 1994). Its antiaggressive effect, moreover, is well established (Jefferson and Greist 1994).

Functional Psychopathology

Thus, the validity of many of our diagnostic constructs is questionable. Moreover, the prevailing taxonomic system defines the diagnostic constructs only vaguely. The reason is that the "choice principle" has been adopted, requiring the presence of only x out of a series of y symptoms – no matter which ones – to qualify a patient for a certain diagnosis. One and the same diagnosis thus covers a multitude of syndromes.

Table 1. Shorcomings of present day diagnostic processes

– Many diagnostic concepts are poorly validated.
– The same diagnostic label often covers a variety of syndromes.
– The comorbidity problem makes it hard to characterize an individual patient.

Add to this that many psychiatric patients suffer from several disorders at the same time, a medley that is often hard to disentangle, and it becomes clear that the need to increase diagnostic acuity is urgent (Table 1).

I have contended that this goal can be achieved by adding a third tier to the diagnostic process, one I have designated as functional psychopathology (Van Praag and Leiynse 1965; Van Praag et al. 1975, 1987a; Van Praag, 1990b). The first tier is represented by a categorical diagnosis; the second tier by syndromal analysis of the psychiatric condition. At the third tier, the syndrome is dissected into its component parts, i.e. psychological dysfunctions, such as disturbances in mood, anxiety, and aggression regulation; motoricity; level of initiative; information processing; memory; hedonic functions; perception and many others. The various dysfunctions have to be assessed, and, if the adequate tools are wanting, they have to be developed.

Functional analysis of the syndrome(s) provides a precise survey of what psychological domains in a given patients are dysfunctioning and what psychological systems do function within normal limits. Moreover, many psychological dysfunctions are measurable in quantitative terms, this in contrast to syndromes or disorders whose presence can only be estimated and expressed in qualitative terms, such as mildly or markedly present. Therefore, functional psychopathology will advance the science of psychiatric diagnosing and will ultimately lead to the equivalent of what physiology means to medicine: the discipline providing an understanding of what the deflections in the psychological apparatus are that underlie a particular psychiatric condition.

Functional Psychopathology and Biological Psychiatry

The functional approach has proved to be particularly fruitful in biological psychiatry. A few examples may suffice. In the late 1960s, we observed a lowering of baseline and post-probenecid concentrations of 5-hydroxyindoleacetic acid (5-HIAA) in the cerebrospinal fluid (CSF) of a subgroup of depressed patients (Van Praag et al. 1970) (Fig. 1). 5-HIAA is the major metabolite of the neurotransmittor (5-HT). There were no particular depressive syndromes or mood disorders predictive of this phenomenon. Though nonspecific on a syndromal and nosological level, this measurement turned out to be specific on a functional level, i.e. negatively correlated with the level of manifest anxiety (Van Praag 1988) (Fig. 2). In addition, a correlation was reported between lowering of CSF 5-HIAA and disturbances in aggression regulation, both with inward and outward directed aggression (Asberg et al. 1976; Coccaro et al. 1989) (Fig. 3).

The correlation between disturbances in 5-HT metabolism, on the one hand, and

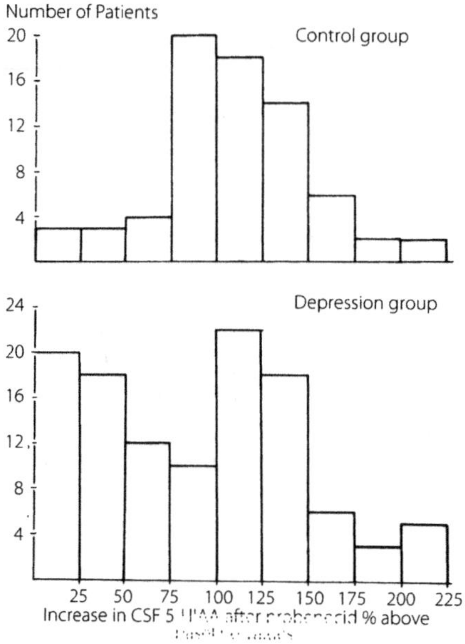

Fig. 1. Increased concentration of CSF 5-hydroxyindoleacetic acid (5-HIAA) after probenecid in patients suffering from major depression, melancholic type (*bottom*) and in a nonpsychiatric control group (*top*). The distribution in the depression group is bimodal. There is a significant increase in individuals with low CSF 5-HIAA. (From Van Praag 1982)

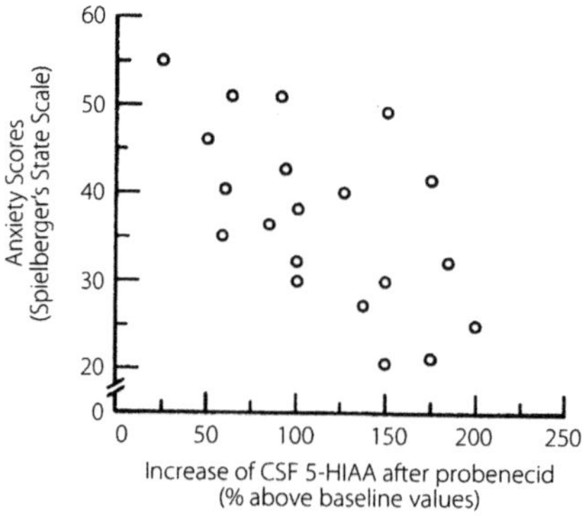

Fig. 2. In patients with major depression, melancholic type, post-probenecid CSF 5-hydroxyindoleacetic acid (5-HIAA) and trait anxiety are negatively correlated. (From Van Praag 1988)

anxiety/aggression regulation, on the other hand, appeared not to be limited to depression but was demonstrable in other diagnostic categories as well (Kahn and Van Praag 1988; Virkkunen et al. 1994). In other words the observed biological disturbances seem to be linked to a particular dysfunctioning psychological domain, irrespective of nosological diagnosis. Psychological dysfunctions are rarely, if ever, specific for a particular diagnostic category. The observed biological dysfunctions seemed to be functionally and hence transnosologically specific.

Functional and transnosological specificity has also been demonstrated for certain disturbances in dopamine (DA) metabolism (Van Praag et al. 1975). Lowering of the

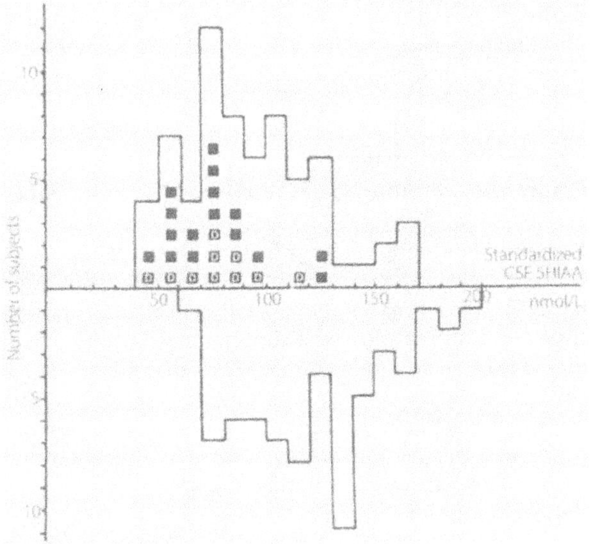

Fig. 3. Standardized concentrations of CSF 5-hydroxindoleacetic acid (5-HIAA) in patients who have attempted suicide (*upward*) and healthy volunteer control subjects (*downward*). ■, Suicide attempts by a violent method (any method other than a drug overdose taken by mouth or a single wrist cut). ⓓ, a subject who subsequently died from suicide, in all cases but one within 1 year after the lumbar puncture. (From Asberg et al. 1984)

CSF concentration of homovanillic acid (HVA) was originally observed in Parkinson's disease. Subsequently the same phenomenon was demonstrated in retarded depression and inert schizophrenics as well. We hypothesized that this phenomenon – considered to be a manifestation of diminshed DA metabolism – is linked to motor retardation and lack of initiative, irrespective of diagnosis (Fig. 4).

Noradrenergic disturbances, as they have been established in depression, we assumed to be correlated with anhedonia. If true, one may expect that the same disturbances will be demonstrable in other psychiatric disorders with hedonic dysfunctions, such as schizophrenia (Van Praag et al. 1990a).

Once more, if a correlation between biological and psychological dysfunctions is ascertained, the former cannot be expected to correlate specifically with a particular

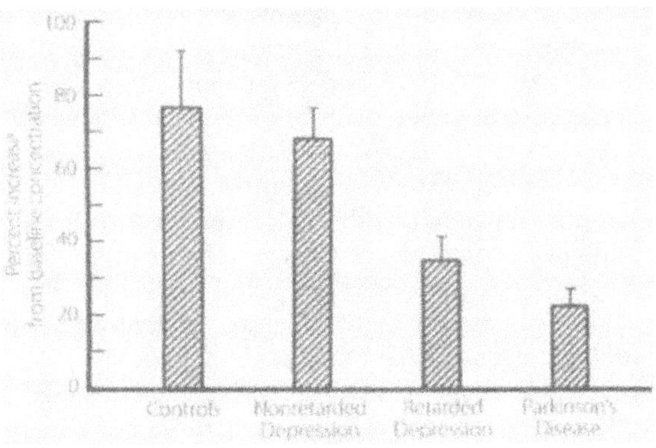

Fig. 4. Post-probenecid concentration of homovanillic acid (HVA) in CSF in controls ($n = 12$), depressed patients with ($n = 11$) and without ($n = 13$) motor retardation, and in patients with Parkinson's disease ($n = 14$). (From Van Praag 1990a)

disorder or syndrome, because psychological dysfunctions are syndromally and nosologically non-specific. Functional specificity of a biological variable implies its transnosological specificity.

Pragmatic Advantages of Functional Psychopathology

Functional psychopathology has the clear advantage that it provides a detailed and in large measure precise map of the psychopathology of an individual patient. By means of this approach the virtually unsolvable problem of characterizing a patient showing multiple disorders simultaneously can be bypassed. Pragmatically speaking, it thus seems to be an essential diagnostic step in executing biological psychiatric research.

One can advance two more arguments in favor of the functional approach in psychiatric diagnosing, both of a more fundamental character than those mentioned above. They will be discussed below.

Verticalization of Psychiatric Diagnoses

A mental disorder is a composite of psychological dysfunctions, mutually interacting in a complex way. The diagnostic weight of the various components is presumably unequal. Some are primary, i. e., the direct consequences of the underlying cerebral substratum, others are secondary, that is derivatives of the pathogenetic process.

Compared to secondary symptoms, primary symptoms are more important and should be the target of both therapeutic intervention and research into the biology of the disorder. By way of an analogy: in a patient with suspected pneumonia, shortness of breath has a greater diagnostic weight than the symptom of fatigue. Before antibiotics were discovered, shortness of breath should have been the prime target of treatment as well as the lead for pathogenetic explorations.

Since the times of Kraepelin, Bleuler, and Schneider, the fundamental distinctions between primary and secondary symptoms have received little attention. The reason is not difficult to guess: for want of methods to study the brain, it was virtually impossible to validate the primary/secondary distinction. Thanks to advances in biological psychiatry and psychopathology, that argument doesn't hold anymore. Our studies in mood disorders are a case in point. They led us to the conclusion that a subgroup of depressed patients exists in whom serotenergic functioning is demonstrably disturbed and in whom anxiety and/or aggression dysregulation are the primary psychopathological features, with mood lowering a subsidiary. If this hypothesis contains a kernel of truth, the proper treatment of such serotonin-related, anxiety/aggression-driven depressions would be an anxiolytic and/or serenic (drugs against aggression) that ameliorates anxiety and/or aggression via regulation of serotonergic circuits (Van Praag et al. 1987a,b; Van Praag 1992b, 1995a). Verticalization of psychiatric diagnoses could fundamentaly change the strategies used to develop to novel psychopharmacological principles (Van Praag 1992a, b).

Attempts to distinguish primary from secondary psychopathological symptoms are a essential exercise for biological psychiatry, since only the former are indicators of the biology of the disorder. Knowledge of pathogenetic processes, in turn, should guide the search for novel therapeutic principles.

Research into the vertical structure of a given syndrome presupposes that it has been dissected conscientiously into its component parts. Functional analysis of a mental disorder necessarily precedes attempts to verticalize psychopathology.

Diseases or Reaction Forms?

I will discuss one more reason of principle to introduce functional analysis as a basic procedure in psychiatric diagnosing, particularly for biological psychiatric research.

Nosology has dominated psychiatry ever since its foundation as a scientific discipline by Kraepelin. Psychiatric disorders are regarded as true diseases, that is, as discrete entities each with their own causation, symptomatology, course and outcome; thus they are clearly identifiable. Biological research, as said, aims at uncovering "markers", and ultimately causes, of these entities.

Mental disorders, however, can be conceived of in a different way, i. e., as reaction forms to noxious stimuli, with considerable interindividual variability and little consistency, rather than as discrete and separable entities. Adolph Meyer (1957) was the first to propose this diagnostic model. The noxious stimulus might be of a biological or psychological nature, could come from within or without, and might be genetically transmitted or acquired during life. The various stimuli have in common that an individual cannot cope with them, physically and/or psychologically. According to this model the co-occurrence of various, discrete mental disorders is mainly appearance. In fact, we deal with everchanging composites of psychopathological features.

In this model the symptomatological variability of psychiatric conditions within and between individuals can be understood in the following manner: Noxious stimuli, i. e., stimuli an individual is unable to assimilate, will perturb a variety of neuronal circuits and hence a variety of psychological systems. The extent to which the various neuronal circuits will be involved varies individually, and consequently psychiatric conditions will lack symptomatic consistency and predictability. For instance, mood lowering is blended with fluctuating measures of anxiety, anger, obsessional thoughts, addictive behavior, cognitive impairment and psychotic features. Between subjects and, over time, within subjects, the appearance of psychiatric syndromes will thus be as variable as the shape of clouds in the sky. One recognizes the cloud; its shape, however, is variable and unpredictable.

The measure of neuronal disruption that a noxious stimulus will induce is, as noted, variable because it is contingent on a number of factors. Most important are the intrinsic qualities of the stimulus and the resilience of the brain. Preexistent neuronal defects may cause certain brain circuits to function marginally. An equilibrium just maintained under normal conditions could fail if demands gain strength. Increased vulnerability can also be conceptualized on a psychological level in that imperfections in personality make-up cause stimuli that the average person can cope with, to be psychologically disruptive.

The reaction form model of psychiatric disorders, if valid, would have profound consequences for biological psychiatry. The search for markers and eventually causes of discrete mental disorders would be largely futile. The farthest one could go is to group the multitude of reaction patterns in a limited number of diagnostic "basins," such as the group of the psychotic, the dementing and the affective reaction forms, each of which, however, would show considerable heterogeneity. As much as it is futile to search for the antecedents and characteristics of, for instance, the group of abdominal disorders, it would equally lack wisdom to hope for the discovery of, for instance, the pathogenesis of affective reaction forms.

Within the scope of this model, the focus of biological psychiatric research has to shift from the alleged mental "disorders" to disordered psychological domains. Schizophrenia, panic disorder or major depression as such, will not be studied, but rather disturbances in perception, information processing, mood regulation, anxiety regulation and impulse control, to mention only a few. A biology of psychological dysfunctions as they occur in mental disorders, would thus be the ultimate goal of biological psychiatric research.

After the World War II, the reaction form model wa abandoned for no good reason, since it has not been disproven. The model offers an elegant explanation for the phenomenon referred to as "comorbidity" by nosologists and would truly revolutionize the course of experimental psychiatry (Van Praag, 1995b,c).

Adopting the three-tier diagnostic approach would provide the opportunity to explore the merits of both diagnostic standpoints for biological psychiatry.

Conclusion

In summary, then, functional psychopathology is an important though greatly neglected and underdeveloped component of the diagnostic process in psychiatry (Table 2). The functional approach provides a much more precise and detailed picture of the psychopathology of a given patient than can nosological and syndromal diagnoses. Moreover, in this manner the unsurmountable problems caused by comorbidity in defining a mental condition can be circumvented. Since many psychological dysfunctions are measurable, often in truly quantitative terms, functional psychopathology provides psychiatric diagnosing with a solid scientific foundation.

Table 2. Significance of functional psychopathology

- Increased acuity of the diagnostic process
- Circumvention of the comorbidity problem
- Quantification of diagnostic components
- Prerequisite for "verticalization" of psychiatric diagnoses.
- Prerequisite for studies of the relative merits of both the nosological and the reaction-form models of psychiatric disorders

Functional psychopathology of a psychiatric condition is a prerequisite for what I have called verticalization of psycho-pathological phenomena, while verticaliation, in its turn, is a prerequisite to target biological and psychopathological research much more accurately than than has been possible so far.

Finally, the functional approach provides an opportunity to investigate the relative merits of the nosological disease model and the reaction form model of mental disorders for biological research in psychiatry. The latter model has been disregarded for a long time; I would rather say, for too long.

References

Asberg M, Traskman L, Thoren P (1976) 5-HIAA in the cerebrospinal fluid: a biochemical suicide predictor? Arch Gen Psychiatry 33: 1193–1197

Asberg M, Bertilsson L, Martensson B, Scalia-Tomba GP, Thoren P, Traskman L (1984) CSF monoamine metabolites in melancholia. Acta Psychiatr Scand 69:201–219

Coccaro EF, Siever LJ, Klar H, Maurer G, Cochrane K, Cooper TB, Mohs RC, Davis KL (1989) Serotonergic studies in affective and personality disorder patients: correlates with suicidal and impulsive aggressive behavior. Arch Gen Psychiatry 46:587–599

Den Boer JA, Sitsen JMA (1994) Handbook of depression and anxiety. Dekker, New York

Den Boer JA, Van Vliet IM, Westenberg HGM (1994) Recent advances in the psychopharmacology of social phobia. Prog Neuropsychompharmacol Biol Psychiatry 18:625–645

Jefferson JW, Greist JH (1994) Lithium in psychiatry. CNS Drugs 1:448–464

Kahn RS, Van Praag HM (1988) A serotonin hypothesis of panic disorder. Hum Psychopharmacol 3:285–288

Lindenmayer JP, Bernstein-Hyman R, Grochowski S (1994) Five-factor model of schizophrenia. J Nerv Ment Dis 182:631–638

Meyer A (1957) Psychobiology: a science of man. Thomas, Springfield

Pecknold JC (1994) Serotonin 5-HT_{1a} agonists. CNS Drugs 2:234–251

Pichot P (1994) Nosological models in psychiatry. Br J Psychiatry 164:232–240

Ram R, Bromet EJ, Eaton WW, Pato C, Schwartz JE (1992) The natural course of schizophrenia: a review of first-admission studies. Schizophr Bull 18:185–207

Rickels K, Downing R, Schweitzer E, Hassman H (1993) Antidepressants for the treatment of generalized anxiety disorder. Arch Gen Psychiatry 50:884–895

Roy M-A, Crowe RR (1994) Validity of the familial sporadic subtypes of schizophrenia. Am J Psychiatry 151:805–814

Strakowksi SM (1994) Diagnostic validity of schizophreniform disorder. Am J Psychiatry 151:815–824

Tsuang MT, Lyons MJ, Faraone SV (1990) Heterogeneity of schizophrenia. Conceptual models and analytic strategies. Br J Psychiatry 156:17–26

Van Praag HM (1982) Depression, suicide and the metabolism of serotonin in the brain. J Affective Disord 4:275–290

Van Praag HM (1988) Serotonergic mechanisms and suicidal behavior. Psychiatry Psychobiol 3:335–346

Van Praag HM (1990a) Catecholamine precursor research in depression: the practical and scientific yield. In: Richardson MA (ed) Amino acids in psychiatric disease. American Psychiatric Press, Washington, pp 77–79

Van Praag HM (1990b) Two-tier diagnosing in psychiatry. Psychiatry Res 34:1–11

Van Praag HM (1992a) Make believes in psychiatry or the perils of progress. Brunner/Mazel, New York

Van Praag HM (1992b) About the centrality of mood lowering in mood disorders. Eur Neuropsychopharmacol 2:393–402

Van Praag HM (1995a) Serotonin-related, anxiety/aggression-driven, stressor-precipitated depression. A psychobiological hypothesis. Eur Psychiatry (in press)

Van Praag HM (1995b) Concerns about depression. Eur Psychiatry 10: 269–275

Van Praag HM (1995c) Comorbidity (psycho-)analyzed. Br J Psychiatry (in press)

Van Praag HM, Leijnse B (1965) Neubewertung des Syndroms. Skizze einer funktionellen Pathologie. Psychiatr Neurol Neurochir 68:50–66

Van Praag HM, Uleman AM, Spitz JC (1965) The vital syndrome interview. A structured standard interview for the recognition and registration of the vital depression symptom complex. Psychiatr Neurol Neurochir 68:329–346
Van Praag HM, Korf J, Puite J (1970) 5-Hydroxindoleacetic acid levels in the cerebrospinal fluid of depressive patients treated with probenecid. Nature 225:1259–1260
Van Praag HM, Korf J, Lakke JPWF, Schut T (1975) Dopamine metabolism in depression, psychoses and Parkinson's disease: the problem of the specificity of biological variables in behaviour disorders. Psychol Med 5:138–146
Van Praag HM, Kahn R, Asnis GM, Wetzler S, Brown S, Bleich A, Korn M (1987a) Denosologization of biological psychiatry or the specifity of 5-HT disturbances in psychiatric disorders. J Affective Disord 13:1–8
Van Praag HM, Kahn R, Asnis GM, Lemus CZ, Brown SL (1987b) Therapeutic indications for serotonin potentiating compounds. Biol Psychiatry 22:205–212
Van Praag HM, Asnis GM, Kahn RS, Brown SL, Korn M, Harkavy Friedman JM, Wetzler S (1990) Monoamines and abnormal behavior. A multi-aminergic perspective. Br J Psychiatry 157:723–734
Virkkunen M, Rawlings R, Tokola R, Poland RE, Guidotti A, Nemeroff C, Bissette G (1994) CSF biochemistries, glucose metabolism, and diurnal activity rhythms in alcoholic, violent offenders, fire setters, and healthy volunteers. Arch Gen Psychiatry 51:20–27
Wolkowitz OM, Bartko JJ, Pickar D (1990) Drug trials and heterogeneity in schizophrenia: the mean is not the end. Biol Psychiatry 28: 1021–1025

The Development of Nosological Concepts in Anxiety Disorders

D. F. Klein

Introduction

The entire idea of an "anxiety disorder" is a relatively recent one. The earliest descriptions of emotional disorders were primarily symptom focussed and often gave what seem to be fanciful explanations by the standards of current knowledge. A classical example is the supposed attribution by Plato of the symptoms of hysteria to a wandering womb. However, hysteria as a nosological category is a late development. What Plato actually said in the Timaeus is that the wandering womb cuts off the respiratory passages with widespread deleterious effects.

What he was attempting to describe was the sudden appearance of attacks of acute respiratory distress accompanied by many other incapacities in women of childbearing age. This conforms more closely to the demographic and symptomatic aspects of panic disorder than current notions of "hysteria," which emphasizes dissociative and conversion features.

Prior to Sydenham, the predominent explanation of disease states was an imbalance of the humors. Normal health was considered due to an equipoise among various organic tendencies (blood, phlegm, cholera, black bile), each of which had their own direction and associated characteristics. Such notions of health as a dynamic equilibrium are common in primitive philosophies, as with Yang and Yin, or God vs devil, or ego vs id.

The important issue is that the doctrine of humoral imbalance implies that there are as many different diseases as people. Further, diseases are not caused by a specific agent and do not have specific anatomical effects or lesions. In such a theoretical framework, the search for discrete illnesses is undercut from the start. Given the ignorance of physiology and pathology, it's not surprising the etiologies proposed were fantastic and misleading. It is to Sydenham that medical nosology owes a tremendous debt, due to his having promulgated an atheoretical nosology, tied to observation of syndrome and course, rather than etiological speculation.

The insightfulness of Sydenham is sometimes missed because the concepts of syndrome and course sound purely descriptive. However, there is a subtlety here, which is that course validates syndrome. Given the extremely confusing nature and multiplex aspects of disease, the development of complex syndromal descriptions became a preoccupation of the nineteenth century. Fantastic amalgamations of symptoms received fanciful names that implied a vague, covert physiology. For instance, the term "neurasthenia" implied a weakness of the nerves, the proposed etiology being the hustle and bustle of modern nineteenth century life, and therefore implied treatment in the form of rest, care and ample feeding.

We paraphrase Hallam [1], who states that, in parallel with medical terminology, psychiatric classification developed broad categories encompassing a hotchpotch of symptoms. Beard, in 1880, made complaints of weakness and fatigue the basis of his new term *neurasthenia* (nervous exhaustion), which included complaints of anxiety.

Freud, in 1894, wrote a paper called "The Justification for Detaching from Neurasthenia a Particular Syndrome: The Anxiety Neurosis", in which he described a group of complaints which have much in common with contemporary anxiety diagnoses. Unfortunately, he appended an exotic theory of causation in terms of the absence, or impairment, of libidinal discharge, considered as a physical process, which may have distracted attention from his empirical observations. In anxiety neurosis were the following features:

1. *General irritability*, e.g., sensitivity to noise.
2. *Anxious expectation*, which fades off into normal anxiousness. This expectation, considered to be the nuclear complaint, is one of danger from a variety of sources. If anxious about disease the term *hypochondriasis* applies.
3. *Anxiety attacks*, a feeling of anxiety: (a) Anxiety attacks can occur without any associated idea or be associated with the nearest interpretation, such as sudden death, stroke or approaching insanity. (b) Anxiety attacks can also be combined with paraesthesias (tingling sensations). (c) Anxiety attacks can be combined with a disturbance of any one, or more, of bodily functions such as respiration, the heart's action, vasomotor innervation or glandular activity. For example, patients complain of heart spasms, difficulty in breathing, drenching sweats, and so forth. In their descriptions, the feeling of anxiety often recedes into the background or is described quite vaguely as a feeling of illness, of distress, and so on.
4. *Variance in symptoms*. The degree to which elements listed in point 3 are combined varies extraordinarily, and almost every accompanying symptom can alone constitute the attack just as well as the report of anxiety itself. Freud mentioned complaints focussed on the heart's action, respiration, sweating, tremor, shuddering, ravenous hunger, giddiness, diarrhoea, locomotor vertigo (a disorientation of the body in space), vasomotor congestion and paraesthesia.
5. *Awakening in fright*, a variety of anxiety attack which can produce sleeplessness.
6. *Vertigo*, usually described as giddiness. Vertigo can occur in attacks with or without the report of anxiety. It also produces dizziness – a feeling that the ground is rocking, the legs are giving way, that one cannot keep upright because one's legs are as heavy as lead and are shaking and wobbling. This dizziness never leads to a fall. Freud carefully distinguishes this from the rotatory vertigo that occurs in Meniere's syndrome.
7. *Development of two types of phobias*. The types of phobias that typically develop are: (1) a type relating to common dangers (animals, thunderstorms, darkness, etc.), which are exaggerations of normal aversions; (2) agoraphobia, often developing after an anxiety attack. Sometimes, attacks of giddiness do not lead to agoraphobia but only to some giddiness in certain places, while alone, in narrow streets, and so forth.
8. *Additional complaints*, including nausea, biliousness, diarrhoea and an urgent need to micturate.

Freud also noted a striking fluctuation in the complaints, with their disappearance in toto for long periods followed by a sudden reappearance.

However, since everybody had his own list of agglomerated symptoms, how could one pick and choose correctly? It was Kraepelin who revolutionized psychiatric nosology by his emphasis on course, that is prognosis. His distinction between dementia praecox and manic depressive disease derived from the observation that patients with dementia precox deteriorated socially and psychologically (hence dementia precox) whereas those with manic depressive illness usually recovered from their illness episode, to later follow with a new episode. Even given the absence of effective tools for amelioration, the ability to make a firm prognosis was still a tremendous step forward.

However, the idea that a discrete disorder implies a particular pathophysiology has been under attack in recent psychologic literature. It is claimed that the very notion of a disorder is a reification, since the notion of a disorder implies the derangement of a normal human psychology and physiology by specific pathological processes. "Reification is the process whereby empirical phenomena, the products of social and historical practices, are abstracted from their context and treated as realities independent of their social origins" [1].

The accusation of reification attacks the notion of a specific pathological process by asserting that since the same phenomenon can be produced in many different ways, that the attribution of specific causality is unwarranted, which leads us back to the idea that there are as many diseases as there are people.

The other covert use of the term reification is to deny a discontinuity between the causes of normal and abnormal behavior. For instance, Hallam [1] says, "Panic may be alarming and incomprehensible, but that is not itself a criterion for underlying abnormality. I will assume that theories of normal anxiety can be used equally well to explain abnormal anxiety."

Factor Analytic Approaches to Anxiety and Depression

Of importance was the growing recognition that anxiety and depression deserved separation syndromally and etiologically [2, 3, 4].

There have been approaches to syndrome formation via factor analysis. Although technically, syndromes would appear to be clusters rather than independent orthogonal factors, it works out that clusters of symptoms frequently appear as factors. The difference is that an orthogonal factor analysis has no implication of mutual exclusiveness so having a high score on any particular factor does not predict the person's position on any other factor.

Two of the outstanding factor analytic investigations are by Roth et al [5] and Fleiss et al. [6]. Roth found panic attacks to be a key discriminator between anxiety and depression.

As described below, the issue of shortness of breath or dyspnea or difficulty in getting breath is of particular consequence to our understanding of panic anxiety. It should be noted that in Fleiss et al. [6] the phobic anxiety pattern included avoidance of public situations as well as palpitations, dizziness, trembling, hot and cold sensations, and difficulty in getting breath.

Similarly Hallam and Hafner [7] found an anxiety complaint factor defined mainly by breathing difficulties and dizziness. Agoraphobic patients obtained higher scores on this factor.

Arrindell [8] also reports a somatic complaint factor which includes "trouble getting breath." This factor was distinct from a factor loaded by a cluster of common agoraphobic fears, e.g., being in open spaces or on the street, or going out of the house alone. It follows that fear of such situations are not rightly tied to a general trait of fearfulness or proneness to somatic complaints.

Agoraphobia Without a History of Panic Disorder

That panic attacks are the regular antecedent of agoraphobia have been established in many clinical investigations. Interestingly epidemiological studies have claimed that there exist a large category of patients who have agoraphobia without panic disorder.

Wittchen [9] stated, "In most subjects with at least one panic attack and agoraphobia, panic attacks as well as panic disorder did either proceed or occur together with agoraphobic avoidance behavior. But it must also be noted that many (almost 50 %) of the cases/patients with agoraphobia had never experienced either a panic attack-like state or the full picture of a panic disorder."

Fyer [10] states: Three out of four recent studies using DSM-III or RDC criteria found agoraphobia without a history of panic attacks was absent in clinic populations [11, 13]. A fourth study reported that 20 % of agoraphobics gave no panic history [14].

The New Haven Epidemiological Catchment Area (ECA) site [15] found that the rate of agoraphobia with a lifetime absence of panic disorder ever was 2.9/100 as compared to a 0.3/100 rate of agoraphobia with panic and a 0.9/100 rate of panic without agoraphobia.

The discrepancy between the epidemiologic and clinical samples is probably due to the definition of agoraphobia employed by clinicians using semistructured interview schedules and DSM-III criteria. ECA data were collected by lay interviewers using the NIMH Diagnostic Interview Schedule (DIS) [16].

The central feature of the DSM-III definition of agoraphobia is fear and consequent avoidance of places "from which escape might be difficult or help not available in case of sudden incapacitation." Avoidance and/or fear must be severe enough to progressively constrict one's life.

However, the DIS definition of DSM-III agoraphobia only required that the subject has found the phobia to interfere "a lot" with his life, taken medication for it, or told a doctor or other professional about the condition. The key inclusion criterion is unreasonable fear of 1 out of 6 possibly agoraphobic situations (going out of the home, crowds, being alone, bridges, tunnels or public transport). The cause of the fear(s) is not addressed.

Therefore, ECA agoraphobia may include those whose fears are *not* centered around helpless, sudden incapacitation (e.g., withdrawn depression, those fearful of crime, or the socially phobic.)

Angst and Dobler-Mikola [17] conducted a longitudinal study of a sample of 600 young adults drawn from the population of Zurich, Switzerland. The one year prevalence of agoraphobia with and without panic attacks were 0.7/100 and 1.6/100, respectively. Subjects were assessed annually for 3 years. On all three occasions, the SCL-90 was also administered. The agoraphobia syndrome was defined using four SCL-90 items: fear of open spaces, fear of bus, subway or train travel, uneasiness in crowds and fear of going out of the house alone. The definition of panic attack is not stated. In addition, to be considered a "case" an individual had to have either social impairment or definite avoidance behavior. Here too, the issue of definition seems overiding.

Horwath et al. [18] have clinically reevaluated such ECA defined agoraphobics without panic disorder and demonstrated that these subjects did not have agoraphobia but rather simple phobia. The problem was that the syndromal definition used for agoraphobia in the ECA had far too low a threshold, thus allowing people with simple fears of crowds, for instance, to be considered agoraphobic. Since simple phobics do not have spontaneous panic attacks, this supposed appearance of agoraphobics without panic was an artifact.

Attempts to demonstrate that the use of the term "anxiety" in various different syndromes does not refer to the same phenomenon was pointed out in an early paper on the behavioral reaction to phenothiazines [19].

Panic Disorder

We [20] have stated: The ability of imipramine to block both spontaneous panic attacks [21] and panic precipitated by intravenous sodium lactate [22] in panic patients suggested that panic disorder is caused by a physiological disturbance.

We considered the evolution of panic. That is, *why* should people have panic attacks associated with dyspnea in the first place? We hypothesized that each person has an integrated suffocation alarm system that decides if they are being asphyxiated, because asphyxiation is a major recurrent danger. The decision that asphyxia is likely elicits intense distress, feelings of suffocation, and the urge to flee to fresh air. Shortness of breath and dyspnea are among the most frequently reported manifestations of a clinical spontaneous panic.

Cannon's [23] ideas about emergency emotions i.e., the "flight or fight" reaction suggests that panic is a type of emergency reaction. However, novel dangers elicit discharge of the hypothalamic-pituitary-adrenal axis (HPA) [24, 25]. These changes have not been observed with panic attacks in the field [26] or laboratory, using lactate or CO_2 [27]. Therefore, the spontaneous panic is distinct from the usual emergency reaction.

Lactate is unique since it comes from only one source to which it returns. Lactate comes from pyruvate during anaerobic glycolysis, which allows continued energy production while an oxygen debt accumulates. Therefore, increasing lactate levels suggest a relatively anaerobic situation. This occurs during vigorous exercise, but panic patients do not panic during exercise [28].

The hypothesized integrative suffocation alarm center compares multiple sources of information. Lactate increment during vigorous exercise is no cause for concern, but lactate increases without hard work would signal hypoxia and may fire the suffocation alarm.

Hyperventilation is clearly associated with panic attacks, although the nature of this association is debatable. To study hyperventilation in panic attacks, we provoked panic disorder patients to hyperventilate without hypocapnia and respiratory alkalosis [29] by putting them inside a balanced plethysmograph and administering 5% carbon dioxide. They were breathing in as much carbon dioxide as they were exhaling which prevented respiratory alkalosis. Before the study, it was thought unlikely that they would panic under such circumstances but that they would panic during hyperventilation in room air.

Surprisingly, the panic patients panicked substantially more in carbon dioxide than room air. This phenomenon was previously described by Cohen and White [28] and was forgotten.

There is 0.03% carbon dioxide in the air and about 5% carbon dioxide in the lungs. The only time one would breathe carbon dioxide during evolution would be if forced to rebreathe ones own exhalations as would occur in a smothering situation. Carbon dioxide increment would then be a leading signal eliciting the suffocation response and the urge to flee.

The panic attack appears to be a three-layer cake. The first layer is the reaction of the smothering alarm system, as if it had received an increment of carbon dioxide, by breathlessness and increased tidal volume. When the control system keeps getting signals interpreted as predictive of asphyxiation, then the panic attack, with its feelings of suffocation and urge to flee, is released, followed by the increase in respiratory frequency.

This provides an explanation for the puzzling finding that hyperventilation is frequently an accompaniment of panic, but that forced hyperventilation is inadequate to produce panic. The components of hyperventilation, increases in tidal volume and increases in respiratory frequency, are complexly related to the stages of panic but are not, in themselves, causal.

De Beurs et al. [30] have recently factor analyzed the symptomatology of panic through continuous self-monitoring of 24 patients suffering from panic disorder with agoraphobia. A factor analysis of their panic symptomatology is particularly interesting. Factor 1, which they have labeled "general arousal", is primarily loaded by sweating, trembling, flushes or chills and palpitations, which are the key features of acute fear. Factor 2, which they label "psychological symptoms", is primarily loaded by depersonalization and fear of going crazy. Factor 3, which they label "smothering sensations", is primarly loaded by fear of dying, chest pain, shortness of breath and choking. It is notable that fear of dying does not load at all on Factor 1 or Factor 2.

This analysis seems particularly relevant to the cognitive theory of panic, which explains such catastrophic fears as the fear of going crazy or the fear of dying as secondary to the development of acute fearful reaction. If that were the case, one might expect that these two catastrophic reactions would load upon factor 1. That fear of dying instead is closely associated with smothering symptoms seems to differentially support the suffocation false alarm theory of panic disorder. That the fear of going crazy is particularly related to depersonalization provides yet another interesting viewpoint on what prompts particular fearful concerns.

The article by de Beur et al. is also relevant to the belief that the panic reaction is simply a manifestation of agoraphobic fear. In this large study, 45% of the attacks were experienced at home whereas only 31% of the attacks occurred in typically agoraphobic situations. Further, one fourth of these attacks occurred during the night or upon awakening in the morning, while the patient was still in bed. Attacks occurring during the night were more likely to be major attacks, which does not fit well with the notion that agoraphobic reactions are a necessary precursor to the panic attack.

Generalized Anxiety Disorder

Gorman [31] states: Generalized anxiety disorder (GAD) is a residual category for anxiety disorders other than panic disorder. The essential feature of this syndrome is persistent anxiety, originally falling within four broad categories: (1) motor tension; (2) autonomic hyperactivity; (3) apprehensive expectation, and (4) vigilance and scanning for at least 1 month.

Spitzer and Williams [32] commented that limiting the necessary period of symptoms to 1 month in DSM-III may make the differentiation of true GAD from "transient stress reactions" problematic.

Consequently the DSM-III-R called for presence of at least six symptoms for at least 6 months. In a recent study by Breslau and David [33], using these stricter criteria reduced the lifetime rate of GAD in a probability sample of 357 women by onefifth (to 9.1%). With the extended duration of illness required under the new criteria, 73% of the GAD patients also met criteria for major depressive disorder according to the study.

In DSM-IV there is a focus on excessive anxiety and worry "occurring more days than not for at least 6 months about a number of events or activities". The criteria list has been simplified to restlessness, early fatigue, concentration difficulty, irritability, muscle tension, and sleep disturbance. Whether there is a real syndromal unity to GAD or whether it is the penumbra of other low intensity disorders is not clear.

Social Phobia

Liebowitz [34] states: Social phobia, for years the most neglected of the anxiety disorders, except among behavior therapists, has recently been the subject of increased attention. Marks and Gelder [35] initially defined "social phobia" to include "fears of eating, drinking, shaking, blushing, speaking, writing or vomiting in the presence of other people," the core feature being fear of seeming ridiculous to others. Defined this way, social phobics were found to become symptomatic and seek treatment earlier, to have a greater male-female ratio, and to have different anxiety symptoms than agoraphobics [36, 37].

Marks and Gelder's original concept included patients with specific social fears (fear of speaking, signing a check, or eating in public) as well as those with more generalized forms of social anxiety (fears of initiating conversations or dating).

Some believe that patients with generalized social anxiety should be classified as having avoidant personality disorder [38], and restrict social phobia to patients with discrete or specific forms of performance or social anxiety. DSM-III asserts that social phobics generally have only one fear, implying that patients with multiple fears or more generalized social anxiety are either rare or should be included in some other diagnostic category. Also, without empirical justification, DSM-III excludes patients from the social phobia category whose social anxiety symptoms are due to avoidant personality disorder, although the grounds for this differential diagnosis are not clear.

DSM-IV more clearly differentiates social phobia from social or performance anxiety following panic attacks. The fact that many social phobics have numerous fears and generalized social anxiety rather than a single fear or simply discrete performance anxiety is also noted. The overlap of social phobia and avoidant personality disorder is also acknowledged.

Somatic anxiety symptoms reported by social phobics may also show differences from agoraphobics. In one series, the social phobics reported more blushing and muscle twitching, and less limb weakness, breathing difficulty, dizziness or faintness, actual fainting, and buzzing or ringing in the ears than did agoraphobics [39]. These symptom differences suggest that panic attacks and social phobic anxiety are pathophysiologically distinct. Social phobics were also found to have lower extraversion scores on the Eysenck Personality Inventory than agoraphobics, whose scores were similar to normal controls [39].

Findings from biological challenge and treatment studies can also clarify the relationship of social phobia to panic disorder and agoraphobia. Patients with panic disorder and agoraphobia with panic attacks show high rates of panic during sodium lactate infusion [40, 41].

Social phobics show a much lower rate of panic to sodium lactate infusion than agoraphobics [42]. As part of a larger study, nine patients meeting DSM-III criteria for agoraphobia with panic attacks and 15 patients meeting DSM-III criteria for social phobia, were challenged with 0.5 *M* racemic sodium lactate (10 ml/kg of body weight) administered intravenously over 20 min. As judged by a psychiatric evaluator "blind" to patient diagnosis, four (44%) of nine agoraphobics panicked during the lactate challenge, in contrast to one (7%) of 15 social phobics ($p \leq 0.03$).

Patients with spontaneous panic attacks are highly responsive to the tricyclic imipramine [42, 43] and the monoamine oxidase inhibitor (MAOI) phenelzine sulfate [44]. Social phobics appear to respond to phenelzine but not to clomipramine.

Subtypes of Simple Phobia

Fyer [45] states: Several lines of evidence suggest heterogeneity within the group of simple phobics. However, at present there are insufficient data to establish separate subdiagnoses.

The most clearly differentiated group are blood-injury-needle phobics. Marks [46] first noted the association between fainting and this type of phobia. Several recent case reports document bradycardia, hypotension and vasovagal fainting in this group [47–49]. This contrasts with other types of simple phobia in which tachycardia and blood pressure elevation are reported and fainting is rare [50].

Animal phobias have a uniformly early age of onset and chronic course [44, 49]. Other types of simple phobias (e.g., fears of storms, lightning, driving, claustrophobia, heights) are also usually chronic but, in contrast to animal phobias, may often begin during adulthood [51]. Marks and Gelder [52] considered animal phobias a separate diagnostic group.

Empirical studies of onset of simple phobias also indicate diversity. Trauma related to phobic object, parental teaching or modeling and stressful life events have been considered causative agents in varying numbers of cases. Many individuals also report no known precipitant. Fyer et al. [53] has shown specific familial aggregation for simple phobia.

Beyond Categorical Nosology to Detection of Functional Impairment

The fact that reliably established behavioral syndromes can be validated by prediction of course, familial aggregation, and response to treatment indicate that certain fairly discrete functional impairments generate this array of associated manifestations and that they are not reifications.

A tremendous cascade of effects intervenes between the etiology of a disorder and its manifestations. Further, there is no neat one to one relationship between manifestations and etiology. In genetics this is referred to by the term "phenocopy." That phenocopies resemble each other suggests that at some point in the causal cascade a similar impairment is produced, although this may reflect quite discrete distal etiologies.

One line of scientific development is to hypothesize what functional impairment might generate a particular set of symptomatic manifestations. Then the deductions possible from this hypothesis allow hypothesis testing. Our current knowledge does not come close to specific etiology although genetic factors seem plain; however, that does not prevent us from hypothesizing about intermediate level impairments. We recently suggested that much of the symptomatology of panic disorder is explicable as due to a derangement of an evolved suffocation monitor in the form of suffocation false alarms.

The line of argumentation goes as follows: Spontaneous panics, as they appear in panic disorder, are usually initiated by a sensation of marked dyspnea. Dyspnea is not a feature of the acute fearful reaction to mortal danger. There is no evidence of HPA activation during either the laboratory provoked or field induced panic attack, indicating that it is not fear. Dyspnea is not due to hyperventilation but rather hyperventilation is due to dyspnea.

The existence of a suffocation alarm system is demonstrated by the existence of patients with congenital central hypoventilation syndrome who do not have a suffocation alarm. Placed in pure carbon dioxide such patients experience neither respiratory stimulation or any sensation of suffocation. Circumstances marked by increasing pCO_2 or signs of suffocation are accompanied by increased likelihood of panic. Low pCO_2 protects against panic.

A likely candidate for the suffocation monitor is the carotid body, which samples from the most oxygenated blood in the body and is stimulated by decrements in oxygen tension or increments in pCO_2 and is synergistically stimulated by both phenomena occurring at once. This then qualifies the carotid body as at least one of the suffocation monitors [54].

One apparent problem with the suffocation false alarm theory is that it strongly implies that suffocation in normals will regularly be accompanied by panic. This seems largely true, as indicated by experiences during cave ins and mine disasters. However, there does seem to be a markedly problematic exception, the slow fading away into unconsciousness that accompanies carbon monoxide asphyxiation.

However, it has been recently shown by Prabhakar et al. (unpublished manuscript) that carbon monoxide is an inhibitory neurotransmitter within the carotid body. Therefore, perhaps the suffocation alarm system does not go off because it has been sabotaged.

This implies that carbon monoxide may be an antipanic agent. We are currently pursuing this possibility. It has already been shown in an extensive set of studies that carefully regulated carbon monoxide can be administered safely to humans. We hope to see whether this safe dosage will suffice to block the panicogenic effects of carbon dioxide in panic patients. This is the sort of unlikely prediction that a good theory should provide. Now, let's see if it is correct.

Similar hypotheses concerning the relation of obsessive-compulsive related disorder to a hypothesized evolved grooming mechanism have been presented by Rapoport, supported by a range of physiological and psychopharmacological evidence [55].

It remains to be seen if similar developments occur throughout the range of psychiatric nosology. Areas such as social and specific phobia seem very promising.

Acknowledgement: Supported in part by PHS grant MH-30906, MHCRC-New York State Psychiatric Institute.

References

1. Hallam RS (1985) Anxiety, psychological perspectives on panic and agoraphobia. Academic, Orlando
2. Roth M, Mountjoy CY (1982) The distinction between anxiety states and depressive disorders. In: Paykel ES (ed) Handbook of affective disorders. Churchill Livingston, Edinburgh
3. Roth M (1959) The phobic-anxiety-depersonalization syndrome. Proc Soc Med 52:587–595
4. Roth M (1960) The public anxiety, depersonalization syndrome and some general etiological problems in psychiatry. J Neuropsychiatry 1:292–306
5. Roth M, Garside RF, Gurney C (1965) Clinical and statistical inquiries into the classification of anxiety states and depressive disorders. In: Proceedings of Leeds symposium on behavioral disorders. May and Bacon, London
6. Fleiss JL, Gurland BJ, Cooper JE (1971) Some contributions to the measurement of psychopathology. Br J Psychiatry 119:647–656
7. Hallam RS, Hafner RJ (1978) Fears of phobic patients: factor analyses of self report data. Behav Res Ther 16:1–6
8. Arrindell WA (1980) Dimensional structure in psychopathology correlates in the fear survey schedule and phobic population. Behav Res Ther 18:229–242
9. Wittchen HU (1985) Epidemiology of panic attacks and panic disorders. In: Hand I, Wittchen HU (eds) Panic and phobias. Springer, Berlin Heidelberg New York
10. Fyer AJ (1987) Agoraphobia. In: Klein DF (ed) Anxiety. Basel, Karger
11. DiNardo PA, O'Brien GT, Barlow DH, Waddell MT, Blanchard EB (1983) Reliability of DS-III anxiety disorder categories using a new structured interview. Arch Gen Psychiatry 40:1070–1074

12. Noyes R Jr, Crowe RR, Harris EL, Hamra BJ, McChesney CM, Chaudry DR (1986) Relationship between panic disorder and agoraphobia. Arch Gen Psychiatry 43:227–232
13. Breier A, Charney DS, Heninger GR (1986) Agoraphobia and panic disorder. Development, diagnostic stability and course of illness. Arch Gen Psychiatry 43(11):1029–1036
14. American Psychiatric Association (1985) Work group to revise DSM-III: DSM-III-R in development (10/5/85). American Psychiatric Association, Washington
15. Weissman MM, Leaf PJ, Holzer CE, Merikangas KR (1985) The epidemiology of anxiety disorders. A highlight of recent evidence. Psychopharmacol Bull 21:539–572
16. Robins LN, Helzer JE, Croughen J, Ratcliff KS (1991) National Institute of Mental Health Diagnostic Interwiew Schedule: its history, characteristics and validity. Arch Gen Psychiatry 38:381–389
17. Angst J, Dobler-Mikola A (1985) The Zurich study. A prospective epidemiological study of depressive, neurotic, and psychosomatic syndromes. V. Anxiety and phobia in young adults. Eur Arch Psychiatry Neurol Sci 235:171–178
18. Horwath E, Lish JD, Johnson J, Hornig CD, Weissman MM (1993) Agoraphobia without panic: clinical reappraisal of an epidemiologic finding. Am J Psychiatry 150(10): 1496–1501
19. Klein DF, Fink M (1962) Behavioral reaction patterns with phenothiazines. Arch Gen Psychiatry 7:449–459
20. Klein DF (1993) Panic may be a misfiring suffocation alarm. In: Montgomery S (ed) Psychopharmacology of panic. Oxford University Press, Oxford
21. Klein DF (1964) Delineation of two drug-responsive anxiety syndromes. Psychopharmacologia 5:397–408
22. Pitts FN Jr, McClure NJ Jr (1967) Lactate metabolism in anxiety neurosis. N Engl J Med 277:1329–1336
23. Cannon WB (1932) The wisdom of the body. Norton, New York
24. Frankenhaeuser M, Jarpe G (1962) Psychophysiological reactions to infusions of a mixture of adrenalin and noradrenalin. Scand J Psychol 3:21–28
25. Dimsdale JE, Moss J (1980) Plasma catecholamines in stress and exercise. JAMA 243:340–342
26. Woods SW, Charney DS, McPherson CA, Gradman AH, Heninger GR (1987) Situational panic attacks: behavioral, physiologic and biochemical characterization. Arch Gen Psychiatry 44:365–376
27. Liebowitz MR, Gorman JM, Fyer AJ, Levitt M, Dillon D, Levy G, et al. (1985) Lactate provocation of panic attacks. II Biochemical and physiological findings. Arch Gen Psychiatry. 42:709–718
28. Cohen ME, White PD (1951) Life situations, emotions and neurocirculatory asthenia. Psychosom Med 13:335–357
29. Gorman JM, Askanazi J, Liebowitz MR, Fyar AJ, Stein J, Kinney JM, Klein DF (1984) Response to hyperventilatin in a group of patients with panic disorder. Am J Psychiatry 141:857–861
30. De Beurs B (1994) Continuous monitoring of panic. Acta Psychiatr Scand 90:38–45
31. Gorman JM (1987) Generalized anxiety disorders. In: Klein DF (ed) Anxiety. Karger, Basel
32. Spitzer RL, Williams JBW (1984) Anxiety disorders. Diagnostic considerations. In: Grinspoon L (ed) Psychiatry update. American Psychiatric Press, Washington (The American Psychiatric Association Annual Review, vol 3)
33. Breslau N, Davis GC (1985) DSM-III generalized anxiety disorder: an empirical investigation of more stringent criteria. Psychiatr Res 14:231–238
34. Liebowitz MR (1987) Social phobia. In: Klein DF (ed) Anxiety. Karger, Basel
35. Marks I, Gelder M (1966) Different ages of onset in varieties of phobia. Am J Psychiatry 123:218–221
36. Marks I (1970) The classification of phobic disorders. Br J Psychiatry 116:377–386
37. Aimes P, Gelder M, Shaw P (1983) Social phobia. A comparative clinical study. Br J Psychiatry 142:174–179
38. Greenberg D, Starvynski A (1983) Social phobia (Letter). Br J Psychiatry 143:526
39. Pitts F, McClure J (1967) Lactate metabolism in anxiety neurosis. N Engl J Med 277:1326–1336
40. Liebowitz M, Gorman J, Fyer A, Levitt M, Levy G, Appleby I, Dillon D, Palij M, Davies S, Klein D (1984) Lactate provocation of panic attacks. I. Clinical and behavioral findings. Arch Gen Psychiatry 41:764–770
41. Liebowitz M, Fyer A, Gorman J, Dillon D, Davies S, Stein J, Cohen B, Klein D (1985) Specificity of lactate infusions in social phobia vs. Panic disorders. Am J Psychiatry 142:947–949
42. Klein D (1964) Delineation of two drug-responsive anxiety syndromes. Psychopharmacology (Berl) 5:397–408

43. Zitrin CM, Klein DF, Woerner MG et al. (1983) Treatment of phobias. I. Comparison on imipramine and placebo. Arch Gen Psychiatry 40:125–138
44. Sheehan D, Ballenger J, Jacobson G (1980) Treatment of endogenous anxiety with phobic hysterical and hypochondriacal symptoms. Arch Gen Psychiatry 37:51–59
45. Fyer AJ (1987) Simple phobia. In: Klein DF (ed) Anxiety. Karger, Base
46. Marks IM (1969) Fears and phobias. Academic, New York
47. Connolly J, Hallam RS, Marks IM (1976) Selective association of fainting with blood-illness-injury fear. Behav Ther 8–13
48. Curtis GC, Thyer BA (1983) Fainting on exposure to phobic stimuli. Am J Psychiatry. 140:771
49. Ost LG, Sterner U, Lindahl IL (1984) Physiological responses in blood phobics. Behav Res Ther 22:109–117
50. Curtis G, Nesse R, Buxton M, Wright J, Lippman D (1976) Flooding in vivo as a research tool and treatment for phobias. Compr Psychiatry 7:153–160
51. Agras WS, Jacob RG (1981) In: Mavissakalian M, Barlow D (eds) Phobia: psychological and pharamcological treatment. Guilford, New York, pp 35–62
52. Marks IM, Gelder MG (1966) Different ages of onset in varieties of phobia. Am J Psychiatry 123:218–221
53. Fyer AJ, Mannuzza S, Gallops MS, Martin LY, Aaronson C, Gorman JM, Liebowitz MR, Klein DF (1990) Familial transmission of simple phobias and fears: a preliminary report. Arch Gen Psychiatry 47(3):252–256
54. Klein DF (1993) False suffocation alarms, spontaneous panics, and related conditions; an integrative hypothesis. Arch Gen Psychiatry 50(4):306–317
55. Klein DF (1993) Foreword. In: Hollander E (ed) Obsessive compulsive related disorders. American Psychiatric Press, Washington, pp xi–xvii

Classification of the Affective and Related Disorders

Sir Martin Roth and Dorgival Caetano

Introduction

Descriptions of melancholia and even the crude outlines of bipolar disorder can be discovered in the observations of physicians in the ancient world such as Aretaeus, who worked in the second century AD. The modern era in the study of affective disorders began with Kraepelin, who classified the functional psychoses into two groups, dementia praecox and manic depressive psychosis in the 5th edition of his textbook in 1896. His concept of the affective disorders subsumed the "folie circulaire" of Falret and the "folie a double forme" of Baillanger, both of which described alternating attacks of manic and depressive mood. Kraepelin's account was more richly detailed. It also included other forms of endogenous depressive and manic illness whether recurrent or single and a wide range of mood disorders such as cyclothymia which are manifest in subclinical form in many cases.

It is noteworthy that his views regarding "psychogenic depression" anticipated some of the contemporary disputes about the scope and limitations of manic depressive illness. He made it clear that the term "psychogenic" in his description of neurotic depression provided no clear line of demarcation from manic depressive disorders. He recognised that the latter endogenous condition was often preceded by stressful and traumatic experiences. But those in a melancholic episode of their manic-depressive illness were relatively indifferent and impervious to the turmoil in their environment. In contrast among those with non-psychotic or "psychogenic" forms of depression even commonplace events provoked responses or even "lively emotional storms". This was an early criticism of the major aetiological significance often imputed to antecedent life events. Kraepelin used the term "reactive" to delineate one particular feature of non-endogenous depressions manifest after symptoms of illness had began.

The controversies which were in progress between the 1960s and the 1980s respecting the taxonomy of depressive illness had their starting point in a classification of the concept of manic depressive psychosis formulated by Mapother (1926). In his view manic depressive psychosis was merely a quantitative deviation from the normal mood of sadness deviating from it only in its severity and duration. He went on to include anxiety neuroses as well as all varieties of depression as constituting the unitary disorder of manic depressive illness. This generated a lively discussion among a number of eminent psychiatrists present at the meeting he had addressed. The most important development that followed was the powerful reaffirmation of Mapother's views of depression by Aubrey Lewis in his MD thesis (1929) and in the three papers devoted to the description and classification course of affective disorders (Lewis 1934a,b, 1936). These views were also expressed in the successive editions of Price"s textbook of medicine published between 1937 and 1966 in which Mapother and Lewis and after 1945 Lewis alone contributed the section devoted to psychiatry.

In a chapter jointly with Mapother (Mapother and Lewis 1937) Lewis described three types of affective disorder each manifest in a major and minor form. Manic excitement had "hypomania" as its forme fruste. Other conditions contrasted in this manner were melancholia with neurasthenia or mild depression and agitated depression at one extreme with anxiety states at the other. "There is no need to try to diagnose affective psychosis from psychogenic depression, cyclothymia, anxiety neurosis, neurasthenia or involuntional melancholia; these are only sub-divisions in which the age, reactivity, severity or chronicity of the condition is being stressed."

It is noteworthy that this unitary concept which implicitly postulated a single etiological basis for a wide range of syndromes was sustained in unchanged form well into the period when the development of electro-convulsive treatment in 1939 and the antidepressant drugs in 1956 had been shown to be effective in some patients with affective disorder but not in others. They had therefore provided a means for submitting the hypotheses underlying Lewis"s unitary concept to investigations that could have validated or refuted them.

The subject of classification of affective disorders is important not only for guiding decisions in clinical diagnosis and treatment in the mood disorders alone. The manner in which the limits of manic depressive illness are defined also carries significant implications for the scope and limitations of the concept of schizophrenic psychoses at one extreme and at the other extreme for the relationship of affective disorders with neuroses; depressive symptoms are a common and in some cases a predominant feature of many forms of neurotic illness.

During the period between 1960 and 1985 multivariate statistical methods were extensively employed to test hypotheses regarding the continuity or discontinuity of the different forms of endogenous and "neurotic" depression as also the relationship between depressive states and anxiety disorders. By including anxiety neuroses within their concept Mapother and Lewis had encroached deep into the territory of neurotic disorder and had obliterated the line of demarcation between neuroses and psychoses. Mapother had explicitly stated that the distinction between them was illusory.

The introduction of standardised methods for evaluating the mentaly ill, specific rating scales and the new methods of statistical analysis made it possible to mount enquiries with a precision and rigour that had not been previously possible.

In their introductory section to the first edition of DSM-III (American Psychiatric Association, 1980) the creators of this new system of classification, which was rapidly to exercise a worldwide influence, set aside some of the knowledge gained in the two to three decades following 1960. The data which had been adduced by the participants in the controversies regarding classification of affective and anxiety disorders were described as having been "inconclusive" along with the implication that they had also been unfruitful. A reappraisal of the main contributions to classification of affective disorders since 1960 will be undertaken in this paper. In the light of the findings that have emerged during this period these conclusions taken from the introductory section of DSM-III deserve reconsideration.

Investigations Undertaken Between 1959 and 1985 into the Unity or Heterogeneity of Affective Disorder

As the disputes about classification and the investigations undertaken in relation to them seem to have been largely forgotten some of the papers that were at the centre of the debate will be summarised before developing the main theme of this paper.

Kiloh and Garside (1963)

The first major investigation in Great Britain was undertaken following some preliminary observations in Newcastle (Roth 1959) by Kiloh and Garside (1963) into 143 cases of depression. They carried out a factor analysis of 35 clinical features elicited in these patients and extracted two main factors. The first of these was a general factor which reflected the extent to which each symptom was related to the entire set of variables as defined by the sum of the 35 features. The second factor was bipolar and accounted for a higher proportion of the total variance in the matrix of correlations between the 35 features than the first factor. The loadings on this factor were very similar to correlations of each feature with the diagnosis made following a structured comprehensive clinical interview. The correlation of 0.986 was particularly high having regard to the fact that no rotation of the factors had been carried out. The second factor was bipolar and could be interpreted as differentiating between the neurotic and endogenous groups of depressive cases tentatively established from the findings of the initial examination.

A total of 92 patients in the study had previously participated in a controlled clinical trial of the antidepressant imipramine. Although a substantial proportion of patients in both groups recovered or improved in response to treatment with imipramine the results in endogenous cases had been significantly better than those in the patients with neurotic depression. This provided independent evidence for the distinction between two groups which also shed some light on the nature of the relationship between the endogenous and neurotic disorders of affect. The results were inconsistent with the view that endogenous depression was merely a more severe form of affective disorder than neurotic depression. It was implausible that the milder and more benign depressive disorder would respond better to treatment with imipramine than the more severe and incapacitating version of one and the same illness.

The results suggested that there was a qualitative rather than a quantitative difference between the two groups.

One criticism levelled against this enquiry was that the separation achieved was due to the omission of cases in whom the diagnosis was ambiguous (Kendell 1968). The diagnosis was in fact reviewed in each case before the initiation of the factor analysis. Only in 92 of 143 patients was the diagnosis regarded as "reasonably certain". In 51 cases the diagnosis was judged "doubtful". They were all included in the analysis.

Carney et al. (1965)

The findings of Kiloh and Garside required replication. There was a need for further data regarding the response of the two hypothetical groups to treatment. It was hoped that the results would also provide a basis for the development of scales for the prediction of treatment response and outcome. An enquiry was undertaken with the

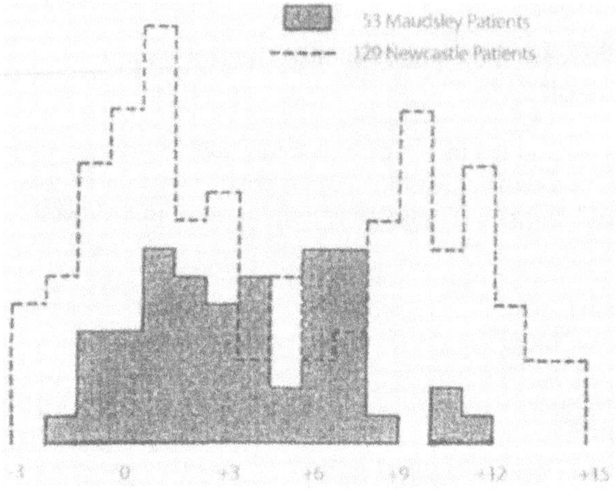

Fig. 1. Distribution of newcastle diagnostic scores. Significant bimodal distribution derived from discriminant function anaylsis of the feature scores on the first factor in the Newcastle study of 129 patients is shown by the *interrupted line.* Distribution of 59 Maudsley patients is superimposed. The comparison between the two curves by Kendell (1968) is discussed in the text

aid of a structured interview in 129 patients with depressive symptom who had been selected as requiring electro-convulsive treatment (ECT) by consultants not involved in the study.

The diagnostic interview was undertaken before treatment commenced. A principal components analysis of 35 clinical features derived from 129 successive patients who were to receive treatment yielded a first bipolar factor which accounted for 21% of the total variance. The second was a general factor which had contributed only 6.3%. This factor contrasted a persistent depressive syndrome with a "distinct quality", retarded psychomotor activity, nihilistic delusions, suicidal ruminations, feelings of guilt, early waking among other familiar features (the typical profile of endogenous depression) with one in which the main features were a long history, initial insomnia, hysterical features, hypochondriasis, irritability, self-pity, a tendency to blame others, and a family history of neurosis; the profile of "neurotic depression". The multiple regressions to be described later were undertaken initially on the feature loadings on the first bipolar factor to achieve optimal separations of the two groups. It yielded a bimodal distribution which departed from normality to a highly significant degree ($\chi^2 > 500$; df = 17) (Fig. 1).

A proportion of patients in both groups recovered or improved after treatment. But the response to ECT immediately after the end of treatment towards improvement or recovery was significantly more often in those with an endogenous syndrome than in those with neurotic depression. The condition of the endogenous patients was judged to be significantly better overall than the condition of the neurotic cases at follow-up at 3 and at 6 months after treatment. There was a high correlation between the factor loadings on the first bipolar diagnostic factor and the response to ECT. But there was more overlap in relation to pattern of outcome than in the distribution of diagnostic scores.

A dicriminant function analysis was undertaken to develop predictive indices for diagnosis and for outcome. The numerical weights of clinical features for prediction of diagnosis and the weights for prediction of outcome of treatment at 3 and 6 months and the multiple correlations under each heading are shown in Table 1. It will be seen

Table 1. Scores ("weights") of prediction diagnosis and for prediction of outcome at 3 and at 6 months derived from a discriminant function analysis of feature scores of 129 cases of depression. Indices for outcome provided better forecasts than those from diagnosis alone

Feature	Diagnosis weights		Electroconvulsive therapy (3 months) weigths		Electroconvulsive therapy (6 months) weights	
	10 Features	18 Features	10 Features	18 Features	10 Feature	18 Features
Adequate personality	134	150		144		189
No adequate psychogenesis	155	128		267		151
Distinct quality	103	093		−028		−159
Weight loss	161	164	429	411	571	594
Pyknic		141	447	526	555	601
Previous episodes	112	081		212		227
Early wakening		076	430	459	402	417
Depressive psychomotor activity	180	098		−370		−255
Anxiety	−140	−159	−427	−430	−340	−359
Nihilistic delusions	249	209		−168		−114
Somatic delusions		058	307	326	354	384
Paranoid delusions		064	211	346	088	189
Worse p.m.		−096	−624	−501	−461	−337
Blame others	−124	−093		−394		−333
Self pity		−044	−193	−205	−092	−092
Hypochondriacal		004	−717	−746	−623	−623
Hysterical		−051	−248	−160	−500	−368
Guilt	094	081		−054		−012
Multiple correlation	0.90	0.91	0.69	0.72	0.72	0.74

that the predictions from the features were almost as good as those from 18 features in each of the three sets of data. A highly significant correlation between diagnostic and ECT prognostic weights provided further evidence for the relative independence of the two main groups of depressive illness under investigation. The binary depression model was therefore validated by the results of treatment and the findings on follow-up investigation. It is of interest in relation to a topic to be dealt with at a later stage that the feature "anxiety" was inversely correlated both with a diagnosis of endogenous depression and with a favourable outcome.

Some Other Studies of Classification of Depression with Multivariante Analyses

These results received further support from replication in enquiries undertaken in cohorts of depressed patients studied by other investigators. Garside et al. (1971) published findings derived from an analysis of 104 patients who had been scored on the Distribution Category Type Scale (DCTS). The distribution on the first component of a principal components analysis departed significantly from a normal distribution and was unequivocally bimodal with little overlap between endogenous and neurotic groups (Fig. 2). Psychomotor retardation emerged as a particularly powerful discriminator. Sandifer et al. (1966) using the same scale derived a closely similar result.

Other relevant studies include those of Mowbray (1969) who refuted Kendell's (1968) inference in favour of a unitary concept of depressive disorders from a recalculation of his ostensibly unimodal distribution. Fahy et al. (1969) obtained a bimodal distribution on a "distinct quality of depression" factor in a population of depressives. Mendels and Cochrane (1968) reviewed seven factor analytic studies (Hamilton and White 1959; Kiloh and Garside 1963; Carney et al. 1965; Hordern 1965; Rosenthal and Klerman 1966; Rosenthal and Gudeman 1967; Mendels and Cochrane 1968) and found "sufficient concensus to support independence of the endogenous and neurotic depressions".

Kendell (1969) considered that clear separation between groups of depression and bimodal distribution of components scored had arisen from biassed preconceptions in favour of a binary concept of depressive disorder. He compared a distribution plotted by Hemsi et al. (1969 unpublished) with the aid of the Newcastle index in 130 patients with the bimodal distribution of Carney et al. (1965) in 129 patients. He describes the former distribution as "perfectly unimodal". It appears on inspection to bear little resemblance to a normal bell shaped distribution. Further examination reveals the distribution of Carney et al. to extend considerably beyond the point on

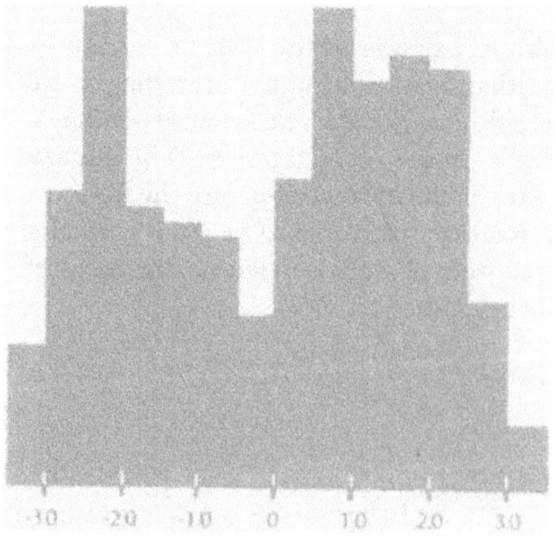

Fig. 2. Distribution of component scores on bipolar endogenous-neurotic factor derived from an analysis of 104 patients. (From Garside et al. 1971)

the abscissa where Hemsi's distribution terminates. There are 51 out of 139 cases with a factor score of 7 or more on the Newcastle Scale in Carney's cohort. In the comparable part of Hemsi"s distribution there are only 12 out of 130 cases. Kendell (1969) did not compare like with like. On the strength of their Newcastle index scores Hemsi et al.'s cohort of 129 patients must have contained a far higher proportion of cases of neurotic depression than the Newcastle sample which contained more than four times as many patients with endogenous illness than Hemsi et al.'s sample. This appears the most likely explanation for the absence of an unambiguous endogenous mode in Hemsi et al.'s distribution.

Another of Kendell's distributions was derived from a multi-variate analysis which yielded a unimodal distribution (Kendell 1968). The findings were recalculated by Garside et al. (1971) from Kendell's, own data. They showed the curves to depart significantly from normality $\chi^2 = 52$, Df 17, $p \leq 0.001$). This distribution related to Kendell's group B made up of 384 patients with depression (Kendell 1968 24, Fig. 2) Hope (1969) judged the balance of evidence regarding their distribution to favour bimodality and the presence of more than one group of patients. Kendell must if anything have been biassed against such a view. Any tendency for his depressed patients to separate out into distinct groups is therefore unambiguous evidence for the binary hypothesis.

Some Criticisms of the Findings Consistent with the Binary Model of Depressive Illness

Dunn et al. (1993) implied that patients in Carney et al.'s study had been recruited selectively by the authors and doubtful cases omitted. All were in fact drawn from a successive series of subjects chosen by ten other consultants as requiring ECT for their depressive illness. One objective of the study was to test the prediction that there would be a disparity in the response to treatment by the groups. In 13 out of 129 patients the diagnosis was considered to be "doubtful"; contrary to Dunn's assertion "borderline" cases were not excluded. Nor were doubtful cases omitted as alleged by Dunn from the discriminant function analysis. In the first step of the multiple regression analysis they were excluded; the weighting coefficients calculated were then applied to the entire group of 129 patients (including doubtful cases). They were all represented in the bimodal distribution.

Kendell (1968) attributed the results of each of the Newcastle factor analytic studies, which supported the existence of at least two forms of depressive illness, as the product of preconception and bias. In contrast, it was implicit that his own findings could be regarded as the product of an impartial and objective approach. The consequences were inevitable. Several of his ostensibly unimodal distributions have proved on re-examination by others to refute or to call in question his unitary concept of the affective disorders. Two of these distributions have already been discussed in earlier sections. The third appears on p. 70 of his monograph. It is reproduced in Fig. 2.

Some 53 patients from the tail end of one of Kendell's ongoing studies had been scored in this enquiry on the Newcastle Scale. The distribution was then superimposed on the bimodal distribution (Carney et al. 1965) comprising 129 patients who had been scored on the same scale. Kendell describes his own distribution as inconsistent with that of Carney in being unequivocally unimodal. This interpretation of his distribution is ruled out on a number of counts. There is a clear dip in the curve at a score of 6 on the abscissa. More telling is the conspicuous dearth of cases in that part of the distribution of his patients' scores on the Newcastle Diagnostic Scale which lies between scores of 7 and 15. This invalidates the comparison with Carney's distribution for it is in this range that all endogenous cases in the Newcastle sample had been located. Of Carney's 129 patients, 52 had a score of 8 or more on the diagnostic scale. But only 11 of Kendell's 53 patients fell within the same range. The difference is statistically significant. It is probable that a higher proportion of endogenous cases would have created a second mode in the upper half of the distribution of his cases.

There is evidence from recent studies that the Newcastle sample is representative of patients treated in hospital for affective disorders. Increasing attention has been drawn in recent years to the under-diagnosis of bipolar and unipolar endogenous affective disorder (Goodwin and Jamison 1990). Patients with unipolar and bipolar endogenous depressions have been found to constitute 35%–50% of patients with affective disorder treated in hospital (Akiskal and Akiskal 1988; Cassano et al. 1989). A similar proportion of endogenous patients in the Newcastle sample (40%) fell within this range. In Kendell's sample the proportion was less than 20%. Such a distribution, which is markedly truncated as it is in the upper half of the range of scores, cannot be validly compared with one which contains proportionately twice as many endogenous patients. Inspection of Fig. 1 (Fig. 17 on p. 70 in Kendell 1968) shows the flaw in Kendell's comparison. It does nothing to invalidate a binary concept of depressive illness.

Some Theoretical Issues in Relation to Unimodal and Bimodal Distributions

Kendell has repeatedly asserted that a canonical dimension separating two groups of patients must be bimodal if it is to confirm a binary hypothesis that predicts at least two different types of depression (or any other disorder) submitted to statistical analysis. This insistence on bimodality as the only criterion compatible with the existance or distinct types of disorder is misconceived. Several authorities (Fleiss 1972; Everitt 1981) have pointed out that, even when two relatively common conditions are regarded as independent on the strength of criteria other than clinical description, investigation with multivariate statistical techniques will usually yield a unimodal distribution of the summated symptom. A bimodal curve is the exception rather than the rule in this situation. It will tend to emerge in most instances only if the two hypothetical disorders are placed far apart by the low prevalence of one or both conditions. A bimodal distribution elicited by statistical analysis of the features of two relatively common disorders such as hypothetically separate forms of depressive illness therefore constitutes particularly strong evidence for their distinct character. The results require independent replication in other samples. But as indicated earlier bimodal distributions have repeatedly emerged from analyses of unbiassed samples of depressive cases. Some of these have been reported with studies that have employed the Newcastle Diagnostic Scale.

It will be evident from the foregoing discussion that evidence in favour of a binary classification of two hypothetically distinct disorders may be derived from a unipolar distribution of scores on a bipolar component. If the mean component scores of the two groups are three standard deviations or more apart the findings are consistent with a binary classification. If there is independent evidence from other variables it strengthens the case for the existence of two distinct syndromes.

Kendell's own attempts to confirm the unitary classification of depressive states assembled a powerful body of independent evidence in favour of the binary system. Hope (1969) concluded after an evaluation of the available data in Kendell's distribution of 384 cases (Kendell 1968, p. 74, group B) that the balance of the evidence was in favour of bimodality.

Follow-up Studies in Patients with Endogenous and Neurotic Syndromes

Examples of corroboration from independent methods of enquiry such as study of the course and outcome of the disorders, their treatment response and neurobiological measures have also been brought to light. The significant difference in treatment response between the two groups in the study of Kiloh and Garside (1963) constituted confirmatory findings. In the case of the Carney et al. study not only was the immediate treatment response different in the two groups, they were also separated to a significant extent by results of follow-up enquiries 3 and 6 months after the completion of treatment.

It follows from the discussion in the previous section that when the distribution of a bipolar factor yields a unimodal distribution in which the two hypothetical disorders are found in separate partly overlapping sections of a unimodal distribution this may provide evidence of an essentially similar nature to that derived from bimodal distributions. Their mean component scores of the two hypothetically distinct disorders have to be significantly far apart and the results require replication. In this case particular importance attaches to evidence from studies of course and long-term follow-up of the hypothetical disorders. Two truly distinct syndromes should retain their separate identities several years after their index diagnosis has been made and their initial course of treatment has been completed. Differences sustained over short periods may arise from transient, contingent non-biological factors. But these would provide implausible explanations for divergent pattern of course and outcomes sustained over years.

Evidence about the questions posed has become available from a study by Kay et al. (1969a,b). A principal components analysis in 104 patients with depressive illness yielded a bipolar factor whose loadings were unimodally distributed. Follow-up observations undertaken 5–7 years after the initial examination revealed a range of significant correlations between diagnoses and factor scores on the one hand and a number of indices outcome of patients placed at the two ends of the distribution on the other. Those in the middle portion of the curve registered scores intermediate between those recorded in patients at the two extremes.

The methods of examination of the patients, the index admission and their allocation into separate groups was described in a first paper (Kay et al. 1969a). The objectives of the follow-up were to compare outcome in three groups of patients "endogenous", "neurotic", and "undifferentiated". A second aim was to study the power of various individual features and the results of a number of structured and quantified methods of asessment in the prediction of outcome 5–7 years after index admission.

Differences between the three diagnostic groups "endogenous", "neurotic" and "intermediate" proved significant in respect of immediate outcome ($p < 0.01$) and Hamilton score at follow-up ($p < 0.05$). Although the endogenous group pursued a favourable scores significantly more often than the two remaining groups ($p < 0.05$) prolonged ill health was significantly more common in the neurotic group (41%) than the two other groups taken together. It was of interest that the number of significant results elicited between outcome and factor score (Table 2) was greater than that between outcome and diagnostic group. Factor scores can take account of differences between patients in the same group and provide more sensitive measures of clinical profile than categorical diagnosis alone. The fact that the undifferentiated group had an outcome that proved intermediate between that of the neurotic and endogenous groups is due to a number of factors. Some pure forms of "endogenous" and "neurotic" disorder enter the middle ranges on account of relatively few symptoms. But those with marked paranoid and hallucinatory symptoms together with

Table 2. Mean factor scores of 104 patients in various outcome classes as determined in follow-up 5–7 years after index examination and statistical analysis

	N	Mean factor score (endogenous-*negative*)	*t* or *F*	*p*
Immediate outcome				
Recovered	47	−0.42	*t*=4.17	<0.001
Remainder	57	+0.35		
Hamilton score				
0–4	54	−0.26	F=5.08	<0.01
5–14	33	+0.26		
15+	15	+0.48		
Prolonged ill health				
Absent	74	−0.12	*t*=0.198	=0.05
Present	30	+0.30		
Readmissions				
None	70	+0.99		
One	15	−0.44	*F*=1.80	0.1<*p*<0.25
More than one	19	−0.02		
Course				
Excellent	15	−0.62		
Good	14	−0.04	*F*=3.66	<0.05
Less favourable	75	+0.13		

A negative sign in front of any value characterises the factor scores so designated as being positively related to some aspect of the outcome of endogenous depression

depression and particularly unfavourable prognosis also fell into the undifferentiated group. These cases were better delineated by the second than the first bipolar factor of the analysis. It is significant that only about 6% of the total group of patients showed a combination of both endogenous and neurotic features. This degree of overlap does not in the case of two relatively common clinical disorders conflict with a binary hypothesis.

There were two features which proved particularly powerful in the prediction of outcome. The first was psychomotor retardation, a feature of endogenous depression which had a very high correlation both with immediate outcome, subsequent course and a low Hamilton Scale score. Its high correlation with a diagnosis of endogenous depression has been confirmed by a number of contemporary investigators (Widlocher 1987; Parker et al. 1990). It also had the highest factor loading among the endogenous features in the bipolar first component in the study of Carney et al. (1965). The other feature "somatic complaints" in the sense of hypochondriacal preoccupations with physical discomforts which were characteristic of the "neurotic" syndrome was associated with a particularly unfavourable prognosis.

This is the only follow-up study on record in which long-term outcome of patients with neurotic depression and those with endogenous depression has been compared with a number of measures including factor scores elicited at the initial examination. The findings confirmed that bipolar factors which yield unimodal distributions of patients" summated component scores may reflect a polarisation of clinical features similar to that embodied in a binary hypothesis. They have the same significance and warrant the same interpretation as bipolar factors that yield a bimodal distribution when the factor scores of individual features approximate closely to the correlations of individual features with diagnosis.

Some Evidence from Biological Variables

Few investigations have been conducted into biological variables associated with the dichotomy of endogenous-psychotic vs neurotic depressive disorders. A number of studies have reported differences between the two groups in respect of premorbid personality. Astrup et al. (1959) has contrasted the well integrated and syntonic personality of those with "manic depressive psychosis" and their relative freedom from neurotic traits with the neurotic and psychopathic personality which often characterised those with "reactive psychosis" (which referred to severe neurotic depressions) and which coloured the symptomatology of these cases. In the Newcastle investigation (Kiloh and Garside 1963; Carney et al. 1965) stable personality was significantly correlated with a diagnosis of endogenous depression. In a study undertaken in Sweden (Kay 1959) patients with marked endogenous features were found to have a history of stable personality and good physical health while the premorbid personality of those lacking endogenous features tended to be unstable and a history of social difficulties or physical disease frequently preceded the onset of symptoms.

It is the genetical part of Kay's Swedish investigation that is of particular relevance. The morbid risk for manic depressive illness in the first degree relatives was

10%–12.7% ± 2.1% and ECT was the commonest form of treatment employed in these patients. In the "reactive" cases morbid risk in first degree relatives was only 3.5%–5.7% ± 1.4% and ECT was rarely judged appropriate.

There is therefore a considerable measure of support from genetic investigations for the separation between the neurotic and endogenous forms of depression achieved with the aid of structured clinical examinations and multivariate analyses of the symptoms derived from large numbers of patients.

In one of the dimensions of Lewis's theory endogenous and neurotic depressions are conceived as more and less severe variants of one and the same disorder. This view cannot be reconciled with several lines of evidence. Clinical trials have consistently reported that it is patients with endogenous and psychotic forms of depression who respond most favourably with antidepressant drugs or with ECT. As they comprise the most severe forms of illness they would have been predicted on Lewis's theory to have a worse prognosis. The findings show that is the neurotic and not the endogenous patients who exhibit on the whole a less favourable response to treatment and have a less satisfactory long term prognosis. These findings cannot be reconciled with the view that the two groups differ in terms of severity alone. Only a qualitative distinction between the endogenous and neurotic depression can explain the available facts.

The Unitary Theory of Depressive Illness: A Multivariate Study of Sir Aubrey Lewis's Data on Melancholia

One of the most clear and important bodies of evidence regarding the unitary theory of Lewis and Mapother which encompassed all mood and anxiety disorders has emerged from a multivariate study by Kiloh and Garside of the case histories which provided the basis of Aubrey Lewis's doctoral thesis.

In the chapter Lewis published in 1937 with Mapother in Price's textbook of medicine three types of affective disorder each manifest in a major and a minor form were described: manic excitement and hypomania; melancholia and mild or neurasthenic depression; agitated melancholia at one extreme and anxiety neurosis at the other. Kiloh and Garside investigated this theory by means of an analysis of the case histories reproduced in full in three papers in the Journal of Mental Science (Lewis 1934a,b; 1936): these embodied the text of Lewis's thesis. The clinical features were described in detail in each case. The symptoms as described in the records are cited in the words used by Lewis together with the number of pages from which they were derived in Table 3 taken from Kiloh and Garside's paper.

Two principal component analyses were carried out by Kiloh and Garside (1963) on the scores of 61 patients (49F 12M) in respect of 51 items. The first three components accounted for almost 25% of the total variance. The first and most important component in each case was bipolar (accounting for 12% of variance) and the items when ranked by their numerical weights as determined from the magnitude of their factor loadings contrasted features typical of endogenous depression with those recognisable as belonging to the neurotic depressive clinical profile.

A cluster analysis using Ward's method was also carried out on the two samples of

Table 3. Symptoms as described in the records of Sir Aubrey Lewis's 61 cases with depressive illness (Kiloh and Garside 1977)

1. Excessive output of talk (pp. 285–287; note 1)
2. Little output of talk (pp. 288–289)
3. Retardation – thinking – poor concentration (subjective) (p. 290)
4. Complains of being muddled and confused (p. 291)
5. Retardation – action = fatigue or anergia (p. 292)
6. Retardation – objective, mild (p. 293)
7. Retardation – objective, severe (incl. stupor) (pp. 293 and 303; note 2)
8. Poor attention (tests of general information, etc.) = "pseudodementia" (pp. 294–295; note 3)
9. Retardation recorded as present (p. 296) and stupor (p. 303; note 4)
10. Agitation – severe (p. 304)
11. Agitation – moderate (p. 305)
12. Agitation – mild (p. 305)
13. Manic features (p. 306; note 5)
14. Delusions of poverty and ruin (p. 307)
15. Conviction would never get well (hopelessness, mostly delusionary) (p. 307)
16. Hypochondriacal preoccupations or delusions (p. 307)
17. Sexual colouring to delusions or sexual thoughts (p. 311)
18. False beliefs or apprehension about sleep (p. 312)
19. Self-reproach: self-accusation (p. 312)
20. Mild or transient self-reproach (p. 314)
21. Ideas of influence upon others (projection) (p. 316)
22. Ideas of reference or of persecution (p. 317)
23. Resentment against others (p. 320)
24. Preoccupations, predominant ideas or delusions of a pronounced apprehensive cast (p. 325)
25. Lack of response to reassurance (p. 328)
26. Dependence or attachment to physician (p. 328)
27. Average or normal adaptation to surroundings (p. 328)
28. Loss of interest or of pleasure in things (p. 330)
29. Depersonalisation (p. 331)
30. Feelings of unreality (p. 332)
31. Disorders of perception – false perceptions or hallucinations (p. 337)
32. Attempted suicide (p. 341; note 6)
33. Denied any illness (p. 344)
34. Denied mental illness but admitted physical illness (p. 344)
35. Loss of weight in spite of adequate intake (p. 349; note 7)
36. Diurnal variation of symptoms (evening improvement noted by nursing staff) (p. 349)
37. Sudden or fairly sudden onset (p. 352)
38. Schizophrenic features (p. 354)
39. Anxiety attacks (p. 357)
40. Neurotic symptoms (other than anxiety or compulsions) (p. 360)
41. Compulsive symptoms (p. 364)
42. Obsessional character traits or frank obsessive symptoms (p. 366; note 8)
43. Gloomy, pessimistic, worrying personality (p. 367)
44. Variability of mood (personality) (p. 367)
45. Sensitiveness, touchiness (personality) (p. 367)
46. Suspicious (personality) (p. 367)
47. Seclusive, shy and unsociable (personality) (p. 367)
48. Adequate precipitants (p. 370)[a]
49. No precipitants (p. 370)[a]
50. Prodromal features before precipitant (p. 372)
51. Sex: M = 0, F = 1
52. Marital status: Single = 0, married at some time = 1
53. History of "depression" in first degree relative
54. Loss of weight (note 7)
55. History of previous or subsequent attacks
56. Prognosis (note 9)
57. Age (years)
58. Duration of first hospitalised illness (in months)

[a] Those scored as neither . . . "were understandable examples of the interaction of organism and environment".

Table 4. Distribution of component scores by cluster for n=61 and n=52. Component scores by cluster fall into two distinct distributions with slight overlap

	All 51 items, first component						25 Endogenous items, first component					
	$n = 61$			$n = 52$			$n = 61$			$n = 52$		
	Clusters											
	1	2	Total	1	2	Total	1	2	Total	1	2	Total
Standard score 2.0– 2.3		1	1		1	1		1	1		1	1
1.6– 1.9		2	2		2	2		4	4		4	4
1.2– 1.5		5	5		4	4		3	3		3	3
0.8– 1.1		5	5		3	3		6	6		3	3
0.4– 0.7		12	12		8	8		7	7		5	5
0.0– 0.3	1	5	6	1	5	6	1	8	9	1	6	7
0.0– –0.3	1	3	4	1	3	4	2	4	6	2	4	6
–0.4– –0.7	8		8	7		7	4		4	3		3
–0.8– –1.1	9		9	8		8	16		16	15		15
–1.2– –1.5	8		8	8		8	5		5	5		5
–1.6– –1.9	1		1	1		1						
Total	28	33	61	26	26	52	28	33	61	26	26	52

61 and 52 patients the smaller group comprisied cases from which nine patients with schizophrenic features had been excluded). The cluster analysis divided the two samples into two roughly equal groups. Distributions of the first component scores by cluster (Table 4) show one cluster consisting of patients who fall mainly into the endogenous range of scores (positive) and another cluster who fall mainly into the neurotic range (negative). The degree of overlap is slight. The results of the component and cluster analyses are mutually supportive. Further the distribution of scores of the total sample of 61 patients departed significantly from normality. A further multivariate analysis was undertaken on the 25 items with the highest first component weights judged by the endogenous features. The distributions of the 61 patients on this first component by cluster (second part of Table 4 were once again almost entirely distinct one cluster consisting largely of endogenous patients and the other of non-endogenous patients. Once again the distributions were highly significantly non-unimodal (χ^2=6.45 df=1 $p < 0.01$ for n=61). Kiloh and Garside's conclusion was stated as follows "... it appears from the data that endogenous depression is an endogenous condition; patients either have it or do not have it – although of course it may vary in severity". This unequivocal refutation of Lewis's unitary theory has been almost entirely ignored in the literature. The unitary theory continues to be upheld by several leading investigators.

The General Neurotic Syndrome

The claim that there are no clear lines of demarcation between the depressive illnesses including the endogenous-psychotic states and anxiety disorders cannot be omitted from any review of the classification of affective disorders. Goldberg (1983) has reported marked overlap between the two conditions in studies of patients in general practice with the General Health Questionnaire. However, Huppert et al. (1989) in studies of a large community sample comprising ten groups of 600 persons each was able to isolate indubitably distinct factors for anxiety and depressive states from multivariate analysis of scores on the General Health Questionnaire. This finding disposes of the criticism of the distinction between the anxiety disorders and the depressive states which has been inferred from studies of large samples of hospitalised and ambulant patients. The unitary concept of depression-anxiety constitutes the main foundation for the concept of "unitary neurotic syndrome" has been recently revived (Tyrer 1989). In Tyrer's model the continuum, in which "melancholia" is located at one pole and "agoraphobia" at the other, there are several breaks in continuity (Roth 1990). The results of a therapeutic trial which were cited in support of the unitary concepts appear to have been indecisive.

On the basis of extensive clinical, epidemiological, genetic, therapeutic and follow-up enquiries the Sydney group (Andrews et al. 1990) have made a stronger case drawing upon personality profile, treatment responses and changes in clinical profile over time for a unitary concept of the neuroses. They conclude that personality and constitutional factors play the major role in the causation of neurotic disorders. They summarise their findings by stating that the different neurotic syndromes are shifting surface manifestations of identical genetically determined personality factors. However, personality had been assessed by relatively crude measures. Moreover as hereditary basis of the neurotic disorders can only be polygenic, the claim that identical genetic factors underlie all neuroses is implausible. Overlap there may be as indicated by the work of Slater (1943). These shortcomings may be partly responsible for the confluent picture of the neuroses that emerges from the studies of the contemporary exponents of "unitary neurotic disorder" (Roth 1990).

The Relationship of Endogenous Depression, Neurotic Depression and Anxiety States

The relationship between the depressive and anxiety disorders was investigated in Newcastle in a number of cohorts of patients suffering from anxiety and/or depressive disorders. In the first instance 145 patients admitted with "depressive illness" or "anxiety state" and using a structured interview that recorded family history, developmental and personality features and a number of rating scales. There were significant differences between the two groups in respect of a wide range of symptoms. Principal components and discriminant function analysis yielded a bimodal distribution which separated the anxiety from the depressive syndromes. Although there was some overlap in respect of affective symptoms persistent depression and episodic tension was characteristic of the anxiety disorders and the reverse pattern of emotional symptoms was manifest in the depressive states.

The findings recorded by independent investigators during a follow-up study over a period of 3.8 years showed that the course and outcome of depressive patients was significantly and consistently more favourable than that of the anxiety disorders (Roth et al, 1972; Gurney et al, 1972; Kerr et al. 1972, 1974; Schapira et al. 1972).

Investigations in a second cohort of 117 patients (Mountjoy and Roth 1982a,b; Roth and Mountjoy 1982) with the same structured interview as that used in the earlier study confirmed the separation of anxiety and depressive states. An important feature was the inclusion of the analysis of scores on seven rating scales for anxiety and depression, as one of the means of testing the hypotheses to minimise preconception and bias in respect of diagnosis. With the aid of principal components and discriminant function analysis satisfactory separation was achieved both in respect of clinical profile and scores on the seven rating scales. Even analysis undertaken on a single measure such as the scores on the Hamilton Depression Scale yielded clear discrimination between anxiety and depressive disorders.

The most comprehensive study of the relationship between the endogenous and neurotic depressions and the anxiety disorders has perhaps been that undertaken by Caetano (1980). He investigated 152 male and female patients with various forms of psychotic and endogenous depression ($n = 66$), with neurotic forms of affective disorder ($n = 39$) and/or anxiety disorder ($n = 41$). The patients comprised successive admissions in whom symptoms of depression or anxiety predominated as also patients in whom diagnosis was ambiguous. The clinical evaluations undertaken with the aid of the Present State Examination (Wing et al. 1974) and the initial allocation to different diagnostic groups determined by the CATEGO programme were a novel feature in this study.

A principal components analysis of 42 PSE items yielded two main components. The first component accounted for 15.4% of variance and contrasted anxiety and phobic symptoms at the positive pole with depressive symptoms at the negative pole. Component I was rotated according to varimax, quartimax and epnimax criteria but the two distributions remained practically unchanged.

The positive (anxiety) loadings of features in order of magnitude were anxiety avoidance, observed anxiety, autonomic anxiety on meeting people, "panic attacks", specific phobia, tension pain, muscualar tension, irritabilitylar, depersonalisation and derealisation. The negative (depressive) loadings in order of magnitude were: observed depression, depressive mood, subjective retardation, morning depression, retardation, early waking, pathological guilt and agitation. The loadings of all these features were significant.

The factor score distribution of patients in the different diagnostic groups as shown (Fig. 3) shows depressed patients concentrated at the negative (depressive pole of the continuum and the anxiety patients at the opposite pole. When checked by the least squares fit method however its bimodality was not confirmed. The degree of separation between the two hypothetical clinical groups justified further evaluation with the aid of a discriminant function analysis.

A cut-off point was placed where the groups of anxiety and depressive states in the distribution of component I overlapped least (at the score of +0.5 in Fig. 3) defined two relatively distinct regions of anxiety and depressive disorders. Sixteen cases with

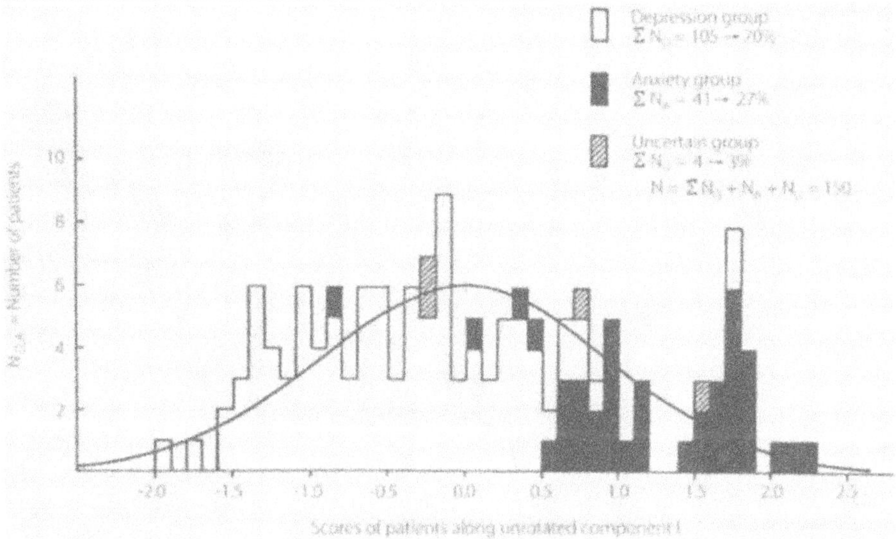

Fig. 3 Distribution of scores along unrotated component shows patients with anxiety and those with depression at opposite poles but bimodality was not confirmed

Table 5. Discriminant function analysis I: standardized discriminant function coefficients and group mean scores

Number	*Label*	*Coefficient*
VAR120	Observed anxiety	.64
VAR018	Anxiety avoidance	.40
VAR007	Muscular tension	.30
VAR015	Situational autonomic anxiety	.28
VAR016	Automatic anxiety on meeting people	.25
OB SYMPTS	Obsessive symptoms	.21
VAR011	Free-floating automatic anxiety	.19
VAR121	Observed depression	−.47
VAR005	Tension pain	−.34
VAR027	Morning depression	−.26
VAR029	Self-depreciation	−.23
HY SYMPTS	Hysterical symptoms	−.17
VAR111	Agitation	−.17
VAR032	Guilty ideas of reference	−.13
Diagnostic group		group mean score
Depressive disorders		(−1.50)
Anxiety state		(3.55)

ambiguos diagnosis were omitted from the first step of the analysis. Table 5 shows the 14 variables extracted by the step-wise procedure and the standardised discriminant coefficients.

Figure 4 shows the distribution of patients' discriminant function scores including the doubtful cases omitted in the first stage of the analysis. The separation of the two

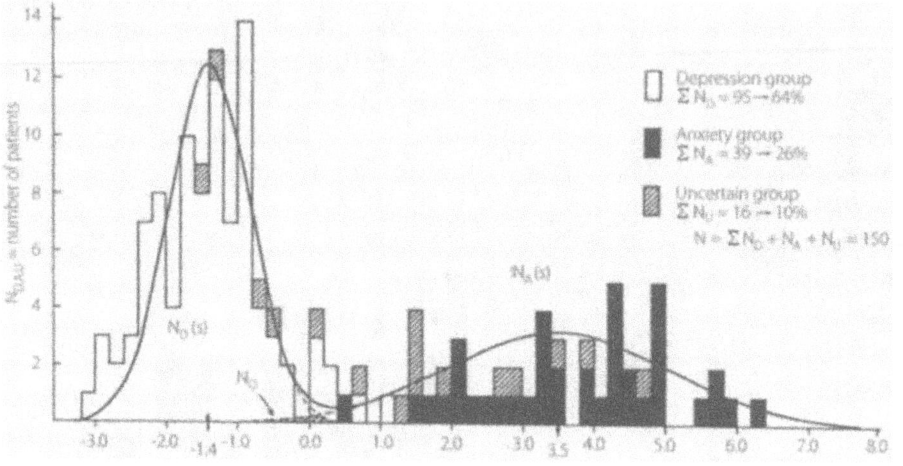

Fig. 4. Scores of patients along discriminant function. Superimposed on sample distribution are curves of mathematically "best fitting" normal distribution

groups is clearly evident. Superimposed on the sample distribution are the frequency curves of the mathematically 'best-fitting' normal distribution. The 'goodness of fit' showed the expected frequency to be very close to the observed frequency as judged by the χ^2 test which showed the difference between them to be small and non-significant. The distribution was composed of two Gaussian curves one with a mean of -1.4 ±.57 the other with a mean of 3.5 ±1.55. The two populations of patients with anxiety and phobic states on the one hand and those with endogenous and neurotic depressives on the other were separated by five standard deviations. The two groups emerge as distinct groups with a small amount of overlap.

A separate analysis of the clinical data by means of a canonical variate analysis and by Ward's method of cluster analysis yielded closely similar results to those described in separating the anxiety from the depressive group and the latter from each other. The canonical variate analysis showed endogenous depressive, neurotic depressive patients and those with anxiety disorder to cluster in a different region of multivariate space with minimal overlap between groups (Fig. 5). The centroids (marked by black dots) are clearly separated from each other and at a distance from the origin of the variates (Caetano 1980; Caetano et al. 1985).

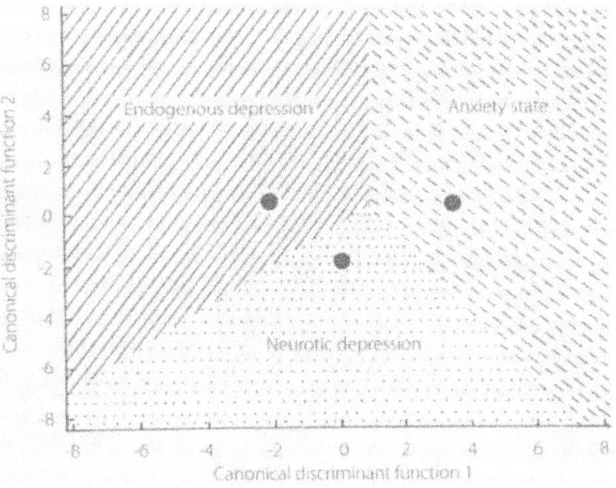

Fig. 5. Two canonical variates served to locate endogenous depression, neurotic depression and anxiety states into three different regions of multivariate space with minimal overlap

The Need for the Diagnostic Concept of "Neurotic Depression"

The elimination of "neurotic depression" from DSM-IV and ICD-10 and the relegation of endogenous-psychotic depression to a subgroup of major depression has proved a source of imbalance and imprecision in the diagnosis and classification of psychiatric disorders. A gap has been created in a crucially important place within the overall conceptual scheme and hierarchical order of the classification of psychiatric illnesses. Unipolar depression has also been effectively eliminated. No satisfactory alternative concept has been included in DSM-III or any other classification. "Major depression" fails to fill the gaps so created for a number of reasons. In the partition of manic depressive illness into bipolar and unipolar disorders anticipated by Kraepelin and revived by Leonhard (1957) both subgroups were originally conceived as endogenous states. Neither had a place in his view beyond the realm of psychotic and kindred disorders.

Unipolar depression needs to be set alongside bipolar depression in the course of diagnostic reasoning and decision making for a number of reasons. Recent studies suggest that of the proportion of the patients who present initially with a depressive illness 30%–45% are suffering or will in due course prove to suffer from bipolar disorder or some kindred condition (Angst, 1984; Akiskal and Akiskal 1988; Cassano et al. 1988). Many cases of unipolar depression may indeed be recognised as such from the transient mild sub-clinical swings into elation before onset or after the end of a depressive episode. Those who regularly suffer periodic attacks at a certain time of the year with fairly clear remissions in between have a particularly close relationship to the bipolar disorder. A proportion of these patients are nowadays treated with lithium carbonate if the attacks are severe or frequent.

In the view of some psychiatrists there is a case to be made for a return to Kraepelin's unitary conception of manic-depressive illness (Cassano et al. 1989;

Akiskal et al. 1989; Goodwin and Jamison 1990). This view stems from the regular and predictable pattern of recurrence, the endogenous clinical profile of a substantial proportion of cases and their favourable response to lithium carbamazepine or other prophylactic measures.

Major depression is not a satisfactory substitute for unipolar depression as at present conceived for other reasons. It comprises a mixture, a "potpourri" of a number of disparate disorders including endogenous, unipolar and pseudo-unipolar disorders. But it also incorporates conditions in which distinct episodes of depressive illness can be defined and which were formerly diagnosed as neurotic depression. The premorbid personality is not invariably abnormal as exemplified by some cases with protracted grief reaction or exposure to other onerous stress such as confinement for long periods in Nazi and other concentration camps.

There is however a certain proportion of patients who, as the original title suggests, have an ill adapted or unstable personality. This provides the setting and one of the aetiological starting points of the irregular upsurge of depressive episodes. What has happened to the conditions formerly described by a number of authors as "hysteroid dysphoria", "angry depression", "the self-pitying constellation", "the chronic characterologic syndrome" and hostile depression? (Overall et al. 1966; Kiloh et al. 1972; Klein and Davis 1969; Grinker et al. 1961; Rosenthal and Gudeman 1967; Schildkraut 1970). It will be remembered that more than half a century ago Gillespie (1929) subdivided non-endogenous depressions into "psycho-neurotic depressions" and "depressions in constitutional psychopaths". In describing the setting he referred to personality disorders rather than sociopathy.

The probable answer to the question posed is that these cases have been assimilated along with "unipolar" and "pseudo-unipolar" cases and some forms of endogenous depression that satisfy the relevant criteria, into "major depression".

Dysthymia does not constitute a satisfactory substitute for "neurotic depression" although this is cited as an alternative name for it in DSM-III-R and DSM-IV. The differences between the concepts are discussed in a response to the critique of the concept of unipolar depression advanced by Bronisch and Klerman (1988) has been published elsewhere (Roth and Kerr 1993; Roth and Mountjoy 1995).

In another publication on the classification of depression (Roth 1991a) an attempt was made to define the relationship between and to integrate new and old concepts. Attention was drawn to the eradication of some important lines of demarcation between different entities as a result of the recent changes that have been put into effect in DSM-III and ICD-10. The elimination of the distinction between neurotic and psychotic endogenous forms of disorder and the substitution of major depression for unipolar depression has contributed to create the areas of confluence between groups of disorders that deserve separate nosological status. In a relatively high proportion of patients agoraphobia, hypochondriasis, obsessive compulsive states, bulimia and anorexia nervosa and other neurotic conditions, there is a colouring of depressive symptoms which is usually epiphenomenal. Notwithstanding this it often satisfies the criteria for a diagnosis of major depression.

Other Continuum Theories: "Unitary Psychosis"

Continuum theories have proliferated in other directions. In a recent symposium devoted to the genetics of mental disorder (Gershon and Cloninger 1994) a number of participants subscribed to the concept of "unitary psychosis" which views schizophrenic and manic depressive disorder as different points on a continuous distribution. Crow quoted the findings of Kendell and Gourlay (1970) to establish the view that the two psychoses are difficult or impossible to separate them on their clinical features. In their first analysis these authors arrived at a distribution which seemed trimodal (Fig. 6) with a peak at the mid-point which corresponded to the "schizoaffective" part of the distribution. In the second sample they obtained a unimodal distribution. These inconsistent findings were interpreted by Kendell and later Crow (1991) as consistent with the concept of unitary psychosis. It indicated no such thing. When summated symptom scores derived from multivariate analyses of two relatively common conditions are plotted bimodal distributions will be rarely achieved. When a unimodal distribution is derived from a bipolar factor in another sample this does not invalidate the first result. Nor can it refute the earlier interpretation that there were two distinct groups in the patient population.

The evidence presented Kendler (1994), who rejected the continuum model, included some data relevant for the present discussion. He referred to nine studies that had examined the risk for affective illness in relatives of schizophrenic patients and in non-psychiatric control probands. Six studies reported no significant difference in the prevalence of affective illness between the two separate groups of relatives. Only two studies recorded significantly greater prevalence of affective illness in relatives of schizophrenic probands than controls (Gershon et al. 1988; Maier et al. 1990).

As Kendell pointed out these findings were therefore more consistent with Kraepelin"s categorical distinction between schizophrenic and manic depressive psychosis than with the unitary concepts. The results in two of the studies were consistent with the unitary concept. But it was only unipolar disorders and not

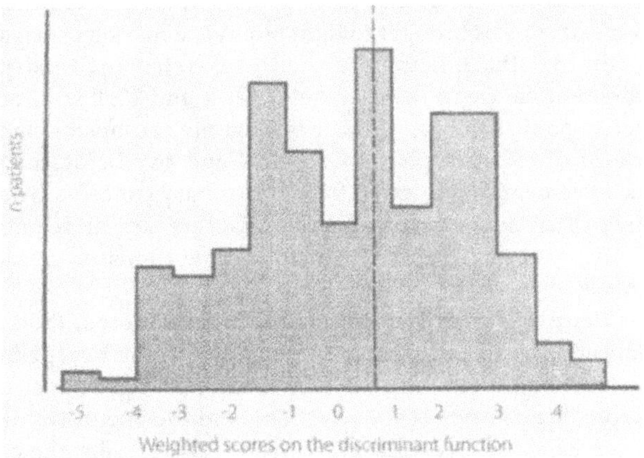

Fig. 6 Scores of 146 schizophrenic and 146 manic depressive (unipolar and bipolar) patients on a discriminant function derived from these patients (Kendell and Gourlay 1970)

bipolar disorder (which should have been increased in prevalence on Crow's model) that was found in excess in the relatives of two schizophrenics" families. When allowance was made for the 5% – 10% of expected error in the differential diagnosis of the psychoses Kendler"s analysis seemed more consistent with Kraepelin's dichotomous model than the unitary psychosis of Crow.

Some points about this issue seem particularly germane here. Not all family investigations yielded the same results as Kendler's. But his material comprised all the methodologically stringent and controlled investigations in the literature and it provided no support for the continuum model of schizophrenic and manic depressive disorders. The second point is that statistical investigations of the clustering of symptoms provided no support for the continuum hypothesis. Erroneous conclusions had been drawn from a unimodal distribution. Thirdly it was not unipolar forms of affective disorder in a strict sense that were found in the families of both schizophrenic and normal subjects. In most of the depressed persons in first degree relatives it was the DSM-III criteria for "major depression" that were satisfied and not those for unipolar disorders in its original specific sense. That substantial numbers of patients with this disorder could be be found in first degree relatives of normal subjects as well as schizophrenics speaks once again for the weakness of this concept as a diagnostic entity and the non-specific character of the disorders identified through its application in clinical practice and research.

Concluding Comments

Unitary and Categorical Concepts

The unitary concept of Lewis which embraced all forms of depressive and anxiety disorder within a single entity has had no consequences other than the work which has promoted its refutation. It is difficult to extract clear hypotheses from corresponding contemporary concept such as the "unitary neurotic syndrome" or the recently reformulated "unitary psychosis" concept (Crow 1991; Roth 1991). The categorial approach inevitably oversimplifies matters but has advanced knowledge of the hereditary basis and pathogenesis of a number of affective disorders and has in some instances brought to light biological markers such as the abnormal functioning of the hypothalamic-pituitary-adrenal system in primary depressive disorders which differentiate them from anxiety states and PET scan abnormalities which characterise panic disorder. It has been mainly responsible for the development of a wide range of effective pharmacological and psychological treatments. No comparable achievements have flowed from the unitary concepts. The lines of continuity between the different forms of affective disorder are of scientific interest particularly in relation to the role of personality dimensions in the development of disorders of affect.

There are wider implications to be considered. If account is taken of the hierarchical order of precedence in diagnosis in the Kraepelinean system unipolar endogenous depression provides an important signpost at the boundary between conceptual territories of the psychotic and the "neurotic" disorders of affect. The term "neurosis" has been discarded from DSM-III. But the concept cannot be jettisoned in isolation without dislocating the conceptual foundations of psychiatric classification. The conditions which "neurosis" subsumes are still there under separate unconnected rubrics such as obsessional, anxious somatoform, agoraphobia-panic disorders, anorexia nervosa and hysteria among others. The view of Angst and Dobler-Mikola (1985) that there are areas of overlaps and lines of continuity between them is not in dispute. But there are also discontinuities and these are more informative and of greater heuristic value. How are controlled therapeutic trials, enquiries into the heredity, biochemistry, molecular biology, neuropathology or imaging of the brain in vivo to be conducted with the aid of continuous dimensions across two, three or more formerly categorical disorders?

In addition to evidence already cited regarding differences in course and outcome of neurotic and endogenous depression important data have come from the follow-up study of Kiloh, Andrews and their group (Andrews et al. 1990). They found in their 20 year follow-up study that, whereas in endogenous depression, personality factors contributed only 1% to variance in respect of outcome, in neurotic depression they contributed 20%. This figure would have very likely been enlarged by estimating the contributions of developmental factors and indices of adaptation from which the personality dimensions would have partly arisen.

Scope of "Biological Psychiatry"

In the psychoses biological psychiatry can be expected in the course of time to discover the underlying causes of the manic-depressive, schizophrenic and paranoid states. These are also the conditions in which biological treatments have achieved some indubitable therapeutic success. Achievements can also be expected with the aid of biological psychiatry in the conditions originally subsumed under the heading of neurosis. When he engages in clinical practice or research the psychiatrist has to widen his angle of vision. In the most crippling forms of illness such as eating disorder and panic-agoraphobic states there are historical developmental aspects to be explored, personality dimensions and the patients life adaptation to be assessed and taken into account in attempts to understand the disorder and its origins. A psychiatrist does not require a training analysis to appreciate that a dynamic dimension is essential for the diagnostic formulation and planning a programme of treatment for patients in this realm of psychiatry. If he omits to explore such facets of the clinical profile he may have difficulty in empathising and in establishing rapport with these patients or to understand them. Such narrowness will be bound to limit the degree of success he will achieve in treatment.

Stringent evidence cannot be offered in support of these views. But the issues under consideration pertain to a large realm of psychiatric disorders in which the application of an exclusively reductionist biological approach is likely to prove unproductive. It has to be faced squarely that the problems and perspectives of our discipline in these areas in particular have a certain kinship with those of the humanities. A North American psychiatrist listening to a monotonous litany of DSM-III axis I diagnoses in place of wide ranging diagnostic formulation on his ward rounds cried out in despair "Have psychiatrists lost their minds?" Jaspers always insisted that in the neuroses and personality disorders biological science has little or nothing to offer; the quest for specific causal factors would prove futile. This extreme version of his concept of neurotic and personality disorders has already been refuted.

There have been significant advances in the treatment of certain neuroses including neurotic depression, obsessional states, agoraphobic and social phobic disorders and some progress has been made in defining causes. Notwithstanding this Jaspers was trying to make a point of profound importance which deserves to be heeded.

References

Akiskal HS, Akiskal K (1988) Reassessing the prevalence of bipolar disorders: clinical significance and artistic creativity. Psychiatr Psychobiol 3:29s–36s
Akiskal HS, Cassano GB, Musetti L, Perugi G, Tundo A, Mignani V (1989) Psychopathology, temperament, and past course in primary major depressions: 1 review of evidence for a bipolar spectrum. Psychopathology 22:268–277
American Psychiatric Association (1980) Diagnostic statistical manual, 3rd edn (DSM-III). APA, Washington
American Psychiatric Association (1993) Diagnostic statistical manual, (4th edn). (DSM-IV). APA, Washington
Andrews G, Stewart G, Morris-Yates A, Holt P, Henderson S (1990) Evidence for a general neurotic syndrome. Br J Psychiatry 157:6–12
Angst J (1984) Switch from depression to mania: a record study over decades between 1920 and 1982. Psychopathology 18:140–154
Angst J, Dobler-Mikola A (1985) Zurich study V: A continuum from depression to anxiety disorders. Eur Arch Psychiatry Neurol Sci 35:179–186
Astrup C, Fossum A, Holmboe R (1959) A follow-up study of 170 patients with acute affective psychoses. Acta Phys Neurol Scand (Suppl) 135
Benfari RC, Beiser M, Leighton, AH, Mertens C (1972) Some dimensions of psychoneurotic behaviour in an urban sample. J Nerv Ment Dis 166:77–90
Bronish T, Klerman GL (1988) The current status of neurotic depression as a diagnostic category. In: Guze SB, Roth M (eds). Psychiatr Dev 6(4):245–276
Caetano D (1980) Enquiries into the classification of affective disorder. Thesis, University of Cambridge
Caetano D, Roth M, Mountjoy CQ (1985) Anxiety state and depressive disorders: separation in terms of symptom-cluster, patient-groups and personality features. Psychiatry 1:513–523
Carney MWP, Roth M, Garside RF (1965) The diagnosis of depressive syndromes and the prediction of E.C.T. response. Br J Psychiatry 111:659–674
Cassano GB, Musetti L, Perugi G, Soriani A, Mignani V, McNair DM, Akiskal HS (1988) A proposed new approach to the clinical sub-classification of depressive illness. Pharmacophsychiatry 21:19–23
Cassano GB, Akiskal HS, Musetti L, Perugi G, Soriani A, Mignani V (1989) Psychopathology, temperament, and past course in primary major depressions. II Toward a redefinition of bipolarity with a new semi-structured interview for depression (SID). Psychopathology 22:178–188
Crow TJ (1991) The failure of the Kraepelinian binary concept and the search for the psychosis gene. In: Kerr A, McClelland A (eds) Concepts of mental disorders. Gaskell, Royal College of Psychiatrists, London, pp 31–47
Dunn G, Sham P, Hand D (1993) Statistics and the nature of depression. Psychol Med 23:871–889
Everitt BS (1981) Bimodality and the nature of depression. Br J Psychiatry 138:336–339
Fahy TJ, Brandon S, Garside RF (1969) Clinical syndromes in a sample of depressed patients: a general practice material. Proc R Soc Med 52:331–335
Fleiss JL (1972) Classification of the depressive disorders by numerical typology. J Psychiatr Res 9:141–153
Garside RF, Kay DWK, Wilson IC, Deaton ID, Roth M (1971) Depressive syndromes and the classification of patients. Psychol Med 1(4):333–338
Gershon ES, DeLisi LE, Hamovit J et al. (1988) A controlled family study of chronic psychoses, schizophrenia and schizoaffective disorder. Arch Gen Psych 45:328–336
Gershon ES, Cloninger CR (eds) Genetic Approaches to Mental Disorders. American Psychopathological Association Series, Washington, D.C., London, England
Gillespie RD (1929) The clinical differentation of types of depression. Guys Hosp Rep 79:306–344

Goldberg DP (1983) Depressive reactions in adults. In: Russel FM, Hersov L (eds) The neuroses and personality disorders. Cambridge University Press, Cambridge, pp 190–208 (Handbook of psychiatry, vol 4)
Goodwin FK, Jamison KR (1990) Manic depressive illness. Oxford University Press, New York
Grinker RR, Miller J, Sabshin M, Nunn R, Nunnally JC (1961) The phenomenal depression. Harper and Row, New York
Gurney C, Roth M, Garside RF, Kerr TA, Shapira K (1972) Studies in the classification of affective disorders. The relationship between anxiety states and depressive illness – II. Br J Psychiatry 121:162–166
Hamilton M, White JM (1959) Clinical syndromes in depressive states. J Mental Sci 105:985–998
Hope K (1969) Review of the classification of depressive illnesses by Kendell RE. Br J Psychiatry 115:731–734
Hordern A (1965) Depressive states. A Pharmacotherapeutic study. Thomas, Springfield
Huppert FA, Walters DW, Day N, Elliott BJ (1989) The factor structure of the General Health Questionnaire (GHQ-30): a reliability study on 6317 community residents. Br J Psychiatry 155:178–185
Kay DWK (1969) Observations on the natural history and genetics of old age psychoses: a Stockholm material, 1931–1937. Proc Royal Soc Med 52:791–794
Kay DWK, Garside RF, Beamish P, Roy JR (1969a) Endogenous and neurotic syndromes of depression: a factor analytical study of 104 cases. Clinical features. Br J Psychiatry 115:377–388
Kay DWK, Garside RF, Roy JR, Beamish P (1969b) 'Endogenous' and 'neurotic' syndromes of depression. A 5–7 year follow-up of 104 cases. Br J Psychiatry 115:389–399
Kendell RE (1968) The classification of depressive illnesses. Oxford University Press, London
Kendell RE (1969) The continuum model of depressive illness. Proc R Soc Med 62:335–339
Kendell RE, Gourlay J (1970) The clinical distinction between the affective psychoses and schizophrenia. Br J Psychiatry 117:261–266
Kendler KS (1994) Discussion of debate. In: Gershon ES, Cloninger CR (eds) Genetic approaches to mental disorders. American psychopathological Association Series Washington, D.C. London, England pp 197–198
Kerr TA, Roth M, Schapira K, Gurney C (1972) The assessment and prediction of outcome in affective disorders. Br J Psychiatry 121:167–174
Kerr TA, Roth M, Schapira K (1974) Prediction of outcome of anxiety states and depressive illnesses. Brit J Psychiatry 124:125–133
Klein D, Davies J (1969) Diagnosis and drug treatment of psychiatric disorders. Williams and Wilkins, Baltimore
Kiloh LG, Garside RF (1963) The independence of neurotic depression and endogenous depression. Br J Psychiatry 109:451–463
Kiloh LG, Garside RF (1977) Original articles – depression: a multivariate study of Sir Aubrey Lewis's data on melancholia. Aust N Z J Psychiatry 11:149–156
Kiloh LG, Andrews G, Neilson M, Bianchi GN (1972) The relationship of the syndromes called endogenous and neurotic depression. Br J Psychiatry 121:183–196
Kraepelin E (1913) Ein Lehrbuch für Studierende und Aerzte, 8th edn. Barth, Leipzig (reprinted 1976 Arno, New York)
Leonhard K (1957) Aufteilung der endogenen Psychosen. (Classification of the endogenous psychoses). Akademische, Berlin
Lewis AJ (1934a) Melancholia: a historical review. J Ment Sci 80:1–42
Lewis AJ (1934b) Melancholia: a clinical survey of depressive states. J Ment Sci 80:277–378
Lewis AJ (1936) Melancholia: prognostic studies and case-material. J Ment Sci 82:488–558
Maier W, Hallmayer J, Minges J et al. (1990) Affective and schizoafffective disorders: similarities and differences. In: Marneros A and Tsuang MT (eds) Morbid risks in relatives of affective, schizoaffective and schizophrenic patients. Springer, Berlin Heidelberg New York, pp. 210–207
Mapother E (1926) Opening paper of discussion of manic-depressive psychosis. Br Med J 2:872–876
Mapother E, Lewis AJ (1937) Affective disorder. In: Price FW (ed) A textbook of the practice of medicine, 5th ed. Oxford University Press, London
Mendels J, Cochrane C (1968) The nosology of depression: the endogenous-reactive concept. Am J Psychiatry 124 Suppl: 1–11
Mendels J, Weinstein M, Cochrane C (1972) The relationship between depression and anxiety. Arch Gen Psychiatry 27:649
Mountjoy CQ, Roth M (1982a) Studies in the relationship between depressive disorders and anxiety states. I. Rating scales. J Affective Dis 4:12–147

Mountjoy CQ, Roth M (1982b) Studies in the relationship between depressive disorders and anxiety states. II. Clinical Items. J Affective Dis 4:147–149
Mowbray RM (1969) Classification of depressive illness. Br J Psychiatry 115:1344–1345
Overall JE, Hollister LE, Johnson M, Pennington V (1966) Nosology of depression and differential response to drugs. JAMA 195:946–948
Parker G, Hadzi-Pavlovic D, Boyce P, Wilhelm K, Brodaty H, Mitchell P, Hickie I, Eyers K (1990) Classifying depression by mental state signs. Br J Psychiatry 157:55–65
Price FW (ed) (1937) A textbook of the practice of medicine, 5th edn. Oxford University Press, London
Rosenthal SH, Gudeman JE (1967) The endogenous depressive pattern. An empirical investigation. Arch Gen Psychiatry 16:241–249
Rosenthal SH, Klerman G (1966) Content and consistency in the endogenous depressive pattern. Br J Psychiatry 112:471–489
Roth M (1959) The phenomenology of depressive states. Can Psychiatr Assoc J 4 Suppl: S32–S54
Roth M (1982) The borderlands of anxiety and depressive states and their bearing on new and old models for the classification of depression. In: van Praag HM, Bruinvels J (eds) Neurotransmission and disturbed behaviour. Bohn, Scheltema, Holkema, Utrecht, 209–257
Roth M (1990) Categorical and unitary classification of neurotic disorder. J R Soc Med 83:609–616
Roth M (1991a) Classification of affective und related psychiatric disorders. In: Horten, Katona (eds) Biological aspects of affective disorders. Academic, New York, pp1–46
Roth M (1991b) Critique of the concept of unitary psychosis. In: Kerr A, McCelland H (eds) Concepts of mental disorder: a continuing debate. Gaskell, Royal College of Psychiatrists, London, pp 17–30
Roth M, Kerr TA (1993) The concept of neurotic depression: a plea for reinstatement. In: L'Approche clinique en psychiatrie (A clinical approach in psychiatry), Collection les expecteurs de penser en rond) vol 3. pp. 339–368
Roth M, Mountjoy CQ (1982) The distinction between anxiety states and depressive disorders. In: Paykel ES (ed) Handbook of affective disorders. Churchill Livingstone, London, pp. 70–92
Roth M, Mountjoy CQ (1995) Comparison and contrast of neurotic depression and dysthymia and its implications for general problems of classification of affective disorder. (in press)
Roth M, Gurney C, Garside RF, Kerr TA, Schapira K (1972) Studies in the classification of affective disorders. The relationship between anxiety states and depressive illness. Br J Psychiatry 121:147–161
Sandifer MG, Wilson IC, Green L (1966) The two-type thesis of depressive disorders. J Nerv Ment Dis 139:93–97
Schapira K, Roth M, Kerr TA, Gurney C (1972) The prognosis of affective disorders. The differentiation of anxiety states from depressive illness. Br J Psychiatry 121:165–181
Schildkraut JJ (1970) Neuropsychopharmacology and the affective disorders. Boxton, Fable Brown
Slater E (1943) The neurotic constitution: a statistical study of 2000 neurotic soldiers. J Neurol Psychiatry 6:1–16
Tyrer P (1989) Classification of neurosis. Wiley, Chichester
Wildlocher D (1987) Intuition and depression. In: Biziere K, Garattini S, Simon P (eds) Quo vadis? Diagnosis and treatment of depression. Sanoti Recherche, Montpelier, pp. 73–89
Wing JK, Cooper JE, Sartorius N (1974) The measurement and classification of psychiatric symptoms, 9th edn. Cambridge University Press, Cambridge

The Ideal Neuroleptic

M. Lader

Introduction

I am very honoured and privileged to have been invited to this symposium in honour of my dear friend and colleague, Hanns Hippius. We first met at the CINP in Munich in 1962. I was a callow Ph. D. student at that time but Hanns already had a substantial reputation in the field of psychopharmacology. As far as I can trace it, his first publications in this area appeared about 40 years ago. One, published in the Fortschritte der Neurologie und Psychiatrie, was entitled: "Zur vergleichenden Psychopathologie der Schock- und Phenothiazinwirkungen" (On the comparative psychopathology of shock and phenothiazine treatments; (Hartmann et al. 1955). The treatment of psychotic disorders with psychopharmacological agents has remained a primary interest of Hanns Hippius ever since. In particular, his inestimable contribution to the establishment of clozapine as the only material advance since the original introduction of antipsychotic medication will remain as a testimony to his clinical acumen and scientific rigour.

I have been charged with the task of talking about the "ideal neuroleptic". This is fraught with difficulty, the first being of one semantics and definition. As Michael Shepherd (1994) has pointed out, the term "neuroleptic" meant "to grasp the neurone" and was originally applied to a subgroup of "dysleptic" drugs in the first French schema. These drugs had two basic properties – to lessen certain psychotic features, and to induce a range of extra-pyramidal (EPS) and autonomic symptoms. At one time it was thought that the EPS effects were essential to the therapeutic actions of the drug but is is now accepted that they are neither necessary nor desirable. Despite this, and despite the popularity of the more accurate and less contentious term "antipsychotic", the use of neuroleptic has persisted. Despite such ambiguities, I shall try to define the ideal properties of a drug designed to treat psychotic disorders, whether called a neuroleptic or antipsychotic or whatever else.

Typical vs Atypical Antipsychotics

The advent of clozapine re-opened the debate about atypical actions of drugs used to treat psychosis in general and schizophrenia in particular. The brief appearance of remoxipride and the continuing evaluation of risperidone have kept the controversy going (Kane 1993). What does "atypical" mean, and which drugs can be subsumed under this rubric (Meltzer 1995)? The common thread in all the definitions is that at clinically effective doses they do not induce EPS. Other suggested properties include failure to raise prolactin levels, efficacy across all symptom groupings in schizophrenia, and no development of tardive syndromes after prolonged use. However, at the experimental level, the definition of atypical generally means inability to provoke catalepsy in rats (Kerwin 1994). The link is the presumption that such compounds will prove efficacious in man without inducing EPS. That this is not generally warranted is exemplified by the long line of drug casualties which have fallen by the clinical wayside, because EPS were induced despite a favourable pre-clinical profile. Yet other definitions include drugs that are non-sedative, block D_1 rather than D_2 receptors or block 5-HT_2 receptors (Nutt 1990).

In my view the debate is sterile and reflects an unfortunate tendency to categorise continuously distributed variables. The important issue, as the clozapine story shows, is the risk/benefit ratio set against the severity of the indication. The ideal antipsychotic would be highly efficacious, without detectible unwanted effects in all forms of psychosis, including the most severe. But let us return to reality and explore the uses to which these drugs, typical and atypical, are put, enumerating strengths and weakness and unmet needs.

Behavioural Emergencies

Before antipsychotic drugs were introduced, the traditional way of dealing with acute psychiatric emergencies was a non-specific sedative such as paraldehyde or a barbiturate or a cocktail such as an opium derivative and an anticholinergic (e.g. omnopon and scopolamine). The usefulness of antipsychotic medication in the treatment of first, acute mania, and then, acute schizophrenia, led to its widespread employment as the drug of first choice in emergency situations. The use of primary sedative medication was relegated to a minor, adjunctive role. This lack of demarcation between an antipsychotic and a sedative function has led to confusion. Thus, high potency drugs such as haloperidol have little sedative actions, probably because they are weak antihistaminics. This lack of sedation is deemed an advantage when the clinician wants to avoid making the patient drowsy (Goldberg et al. 1989). However, in most cases, the patient needs quietening, especially if he is hostile and potentially violent. Using a drug like chlorpromazine or thioridazine in high doses is illogical as one is relying to a substantial extent on their antihistaminic sedative actions. And there are more effective sedatives than antihistamines!

Furthermore, large doses of antipsychotics, so-called rapid tranquillisation, is not without its unwanted effects and indeed dangers. Orthostatic hypotension following peripheral alpha-adrenergic blockade can be a problem, as can anticholinergic effects. Acute dystonias are common with an incidence of at least 10 % during the first 24 h after rapid tranquillisation (Dubin et al. 1985). Rapid escalation of dose can lead to the neuroleptic malignant syndrome (Gratz and Simpson 1994) but this is not usually a problem after single-dose interventions. Seizures may, however, occur.

The most catastrophic adverse event is sudden death and this has been causing increasing concern. Although some uncertainty surrounds the involvement of antipsychotic drug treatment (Task Force 1987), a recent evaluation of post-mortem drug concentrations in a small series of young people on antipsychotic medication dying suddenly concluded that in most cases a definite link could be established (Jusic and Lader 1994). Indeed, suspicion is pharmacologically justified as potentially toxic effects of phenothiazines on the heart have long been known. This may be due to actions on cation channels rather than on dopamine receptors. The struggling patient may be at increased risk, perhaps the release of adrenaline sensitising the heart. Conversely, the oversedated patient can develop respiratory depression and pneumonia.

Because of these various problems, attention has shifted back to sedatives, particularly the safer modern ones, the benzodiazepines (Lingjaerde 1991). The main danger is respiratory depression, and laryngeal spasm may rarely occur. Unlike the antipsychotic drugs, a specific antidote for the benzodiazepines is available, and flumazenil can quickly reverse unwanted adverse effects.

The combination of an antipsychotic drug and a benzodiazepine is often used as the preferred medication to quieten the disturbed patient. In one survey in my hospital, haloperidol was combined with diazepam, 10 mg of each being favoured (Pilowsky et al. 1992). Given intravenously, the quietening effect was very rapid but several attendants are needed to restrain the patient sufficiently to ensure a clean venepuncture. Some practitioners prefer lorazepam intramuscularly because of the lesser problems of injection but diazepam is unreliable by this mode of administration.

Thus, the ideal neuroleptic would have prompt efficacy in containing the acutely disturbed patient, without untoward effects and certainly without the rare but extremely tragic sudden deaths. Ease of administration is another necessity. However, I believe it unrealistic to expect compounds to be effective both in combating the psychopathological symptoms of psychosis on repeated administration and in quietening the behavioural disturbance on single administration. Meanwhile, I believe that acute tranquillisation should concentrate on primary sedation with a benzodiazepine.

Acute Treatment

Although chlorpromazine was first tried in manic patients, it eventually became established as the choice in schizophrenia, and I will confine my discussion to that indication.

For many sufferers, schizophrenia is a chronic relapsing and remitting condition. The typical clinical course is of stretches of relative stability and adaptation punctuated by periods of acute relapse, deterioration and social decompensation. The purposes of maintenance medication which I shall review later is to prevent such relapses. Nevertheless, relapse is common, sometimes despite continued medication, sometimes following inadequate compliance. Whatever the reasons (and they mostly remain obscure), the relapse can present substantial treatment problems and vastly complicate the long term management of the individual afflicted with schizophrenia.

The acute relapse is generally characterised by an increase in positive symptoms such as delusions and hallucinations, thought disorder and agitation. Behavioural disorganisation is common. Negative symptoms may increase with extreme social withdrawal and inertia, and even mutism. The increase in negative symptoms may be interpreted as an attempt by the patient to control intolerable positive symptoms or they may appear to be primary, particularly in the later stages of the illness.

The efficacy of all the conventional antipsychotic drugs is limited, with some patients perhaps up to a third remaining ill, tormented by their voices, agitated or unpredictably aggressive. Dosages are racked up in an increasing atmosphere of tight-lipped desperation. If in the community, the family or the warden of the hostel find themselves drawn increasingly into the maelstrom of the patient's psychotic behaviour. In hospital, the patient needs special attention or intensive supervision, putting strains on the usually inadequately-staffed nursing and other services. This limited efficacy is common to all the typical neuroleptics, almost all comparative trials failing to uncover differences. However, the clinical impression exists that some patients do better on one drug than another. Unfortunately, the natural history of drug medication in schizophrenia is of many drugs being tried, sometimes in succession but too often in combination when it is impossible to disentangle where to assign credit for any apparent efficacy.

As with other classes of psychotropic drugs, attempts have been made to optimise drug treatment using pharmacokinetic measures (Balant-Gorgia et al. 1993). The early work concentrated on chlorpromazine, an unfortunate choice because of the complexity of its metabolism: no reliable relationship was found between bodily concentrations and response. More recent work with haloperidol has indicated a curvilinear relationship, both low and high levels being associated with a poor response (e.g. Van Putten et al. 1992; Volavka et al. 1992). Wirshing et al. (1995) advocate plasma drug concentration monitoring when the patient fails to respond; when side effects are difficult to distinguish from features of the illness; when drug combinations are used; in the young, the old and the infirm; and in suspected poor compliance.

Functional neuroimaging takes this area of research one (major) step forward by exploring the relationship between receptor occupancy and response. By and large, this relationship is much stronger for EPS than for efficacy (e.g. Farde et al. 1992), which is not surprising as the dopamine receptors are mainly visualised in the basal ganglia.

Where neuroleptic drugs do differ in major ways is in respect to their side-effect profile. This topic has been reviewed many times and proves a fertile area for research because of the complex pharmacology of these drugs. The choice of typical antipsychotic drug generally depends on the tolerability of that drug to that patient. Some patients find akathisia intolerable, others sedation. But the problems of side effects are much more important in long term treatment.

The atypical compound, clozapine, has thrown up many questions concerning the treatment of schizophrenia and other psychoses. It is the only antipsychotic with proven efficacy in otherwise treatment-resistant patients, although some new contenders are jockeying for position (Meltzer 1995). The history of the development of clozapine has been well-documented, not least by Hanns Hippius himself (Hippius 1989). But what intrigues me is the plethora of unusual qualities (Lader 1992). Thus:

1. It is effective in 30 % – 60 % of otherwise treatment-resistant schizophrenics.
2. It has some efficacy against negative as well as positive symptoms.
3. The extrapyramidal side-effects are usually mild.
4. There is little or no tardive dyskinesia.
5. There is no marked elevation of prolactin.
6. Hypersalivation is a frequent side-effect.
7. There is a 1 % – 2 % incidence of granulocytopenia.

Are these properties linked? Occum's razor principle dictates that we must assume that, but clozapine may possess more than one unique property which would explain that concentrating on one atypical feature at a time has so far not resulted in a compound with similar efficacy and few unwanted effects but without the risk of blood dyscrasia.

Long-Term Treatment

The long term treatment of schizophrenia patients with antipsychotic drugs is designed to minimize chronic symptoms, both positive and negative and to prevent acute exacerbations of illness (Csernansky and Newcomer 1995). However, these two goals are neither separate nor closely linked. Different courses of illness are seen in different patients, some being relatively normal but with horrendous episodes of acute illness, others remaining disturbed and symptomatic all the time with apparent random fluctuations in severity. A secondary issue is the minimization of side effects. This goal is closely linked to the others via the mediating mechanism of compliance.

Table 1. Factors influencing relapse in schizophrenic patients

Illness
Insidious onset
Negative symptoms
Thought disorder and disorganization
Male, young
Poor response to treatment
Drug treatment
Inadequate dosage
Intolerable side effects
Idiosyncratic responses
Personal
Poor compliance
Substance and alcohol abuse
Poor coping abilities
Social/occupational
Social isolation
Major life events
Unemployment
High expressed emotion

It is well established that patients with the relapsing form of schizophrenia tend to maintain their likelihood of further relapses. For example, the mean rate of psychotic relapse in patients in apparent remission or partial remission maintained on placebo is as high as 60%–80% within 12 months (Kane and Lieberman 1987). This rate is at least halved by regular taking of antipsychotic medication (Davis 1985). The factors which predispose to relapse are various (Lader 1995). They can be divided into several categories which include illness, drug treatment, personal and social/occupational (Table 1).

The unwanted effects of antipsychotic medication are multifarious and have been listed many times (e.g. Bristow and Hirsch 1993). They comprise acute neuromuscular problems such as dystonia, akathisia, parkinsonism and the neuroleptic malignant syndrome; long term neuromuscular effects such as tardive dystonia and tardive dyskinesia; endocrine and metabolic complications including hyperprolactinaemia and obesity; cardiovascular effects such as postural hypotension, and cardiac arrhythmias; central nervous system problems such as seizures, cognitive impairment and perhaps a pseudo-depressive state; and many other effects on the blood, skin, eye and liver.

The practical clinical importance of these side-effects range from trivial inconveniences such as mild dry mouth to life-threatening untoward events such as agranulocytosis. In between these extremes, side effects can be ranked according to their degree of "unwantedness". However, this rank order will differ according to the viewpoint of the assessor. The doctor may have an attitude different to that of the patient. Thus, the doctor will rank cardiac arrhythmia as highly undesirable; the patient may be unaware of it. Conversely, the carer may be irritated by the fuss made by the patient over a subjective symptom such as sedation. While we are capable of quantifying the risks involved in side effects, we have little knowledge of patients' views on their medication. This neglect has resulted in a poor understanding of the factors which lead to non-compliance with the greatly increased risk of relapse.

One relevant study is that of Windgassen (1992). He questioned 61 schizophrenic patients on the effects which they ascribed to their neuroleptic medication. Half the patients commented adversely on sedation, 19 described akinesia and 11 complained of problems thinking or concentrating. Among physical side effects, 10 complained of salivation disorders, and 10 of visual disturbances. An interesting section in the paper probes the phenomenology of the sedation. It is not simply drowsiness, i.e. a feeling of wanting to go to sleep. Rather, it is described as feeling leaden, as malaise, as anxiety with suppression, as being switched off. This has been dubbed the "zombie" effect (Lader 1994). The entire syndrome has been noticed for many years and more recently has been called the neuroleptic-induced deficit syndrome) (NIDS) (Lader and Lewander 1994).

The importance of these unwanted effects resides not only in the impairment of the patients' quality of life but also in compliance issues. Some overt refusal of medication reflects severe psychopathology and negative attitudes towards hospital and treatment. However, about a third of patients refusing medication in one large scale study gave medication side effects as the reason and 12% avowed the treatment to be ineffective (Hoge et al. 1990). It would be expected that covert non- or poor compliance would be even higher especially in patients outside hospital. Administration of antiparkinsonian medication has been claimed to improve compliance with neuroleptic medication (Van Putten 1974).

The whole topic of subjective side effects of neuroleptic medication is very convoluted. The main factors are the schizophrenic illness with its pleomorphic phenomenology, the variable course of the illness, superadded disorders such as depressive phases during resolution of a relapse, pseudoparkinsonism and akathisia as EPS side effects of antipsychotic medication, and dysphoric sedation as another type of side effect. Attempts to disentangle these elements, for example, by discontinuing medication, have shown features common to negative symptoms and depression (Newcomer et al. 1990) and to pseudoparkinsonism (Prosser et al. 1987).

Laboratory testing of cognitive and neuropsychological function has revealed quite selective effects of antipsychotic medication (Cassens et al. 1990). A complicating factor is the impairment of motor function due to EPS. This has to be very carefully evaluated when exploring possible advantages of atypical neuroleptics such as clozapine and risperidone. The low incidence of EPS may be confounded with and by a lack of effect on central cognitive functioning (e.g. Buchanan et al. 1994).

A final point concerns the usefulness of depot antipsychotic drugs. A coruscating review by John Davis and his colleagues (1994) concluded that depot medication is indicated to achieve continuous treatment in both the admittedly non-compliant patient and in those with frequent relapses, who must be assumed to be non-compliers.

From the above, the properties of the ideal long term neuroleptic seem clear. It should have enhanced efficacy, preventing relapses with all their consequent psychosocial disruption, and controlling ongoing positive, negative and disorganisational symptoms. It should have minimal side effects and those that are present should not compromise compliance. Long term medication should be formulated to be convenient and flexible but still, as with depot medications, providing an effective drug concentration in the patient who is poorly compliant for whatever reason.

Other Considerations

Many other factors govern our consideration of the attributes of an ideal neuroleptic. Let me focus on just two. Drug and alcohol abuse among psychiatric patients has been increasing rapidly, although probably no more so than in the general population. However, it seems now that up to a half of newly presenting schizophrenic patients in the USA have substance abuse problems (Regier et al. 1990). This excludes those whose psychotic phenomena are only present during periods of drug-taking. The relationship between the two forms of morbidity is uncertain: this problem dates back a long time, for example, to amphetamine psychosis and subsequent schizophrenia. Does the alcohol or drug-taking cause the psychosis, bring it forward in time, or is it a symptom of disintegrating normal behaviour patterns? It is not clear whether the clinical course is subsequently different in the substance-abusing schizophrenics or if they are prone to more violence like their non-psychotic peers (Smith and Hucker 1994).

The link between substance and schizophrenia is of more than clinical interest only. Dopamine is known to be involved in mechanisms of reward and of psychotic behaviour. Less well-established is the role of serotonin in consummatory behaviour and in schizophrenia. Thus, the more theoretical aspects of the conjunction of psychosis and substance abuse might also give pointers to one of the properties of an ideal hypnotic, namely, to be effective as both an antipsychotic and in lessening usage of alcohol and drugs of abuse.

The final topic I wish to mention concerns a particular interest of mine, the combination of drug and non-drug methods of management of the schizophrenic patient. A large and distinguished body of work on social aspects of psychosis has led to the development of various techniques to optimize the environment of the patient.

Occupational problems have been addressed by setting up rehabilitation workshops with carefully graded types of work and by counselling patients on appropriate occupations and careers. Residential hostels with carefully graded degrees of supervision have been set up and placement in this system must be finely judged. The family constellation is explored, especially with respect to the balance of support and pressure placed on the patient, and note is taken of the amount of interaction which takes place within the family structure. Where the family situation is deemed unsatisfactory, family intervention has become a standard method of management. A recent review examined over 300 citations and found six randomized controlled trials involving 350 patients which were then incorporated into a meta-analysis (De Jesus Mari and Streiner 1994). The likelihood of relapse was significantly reduced in the experimental as compared with the control group. Compliance with drug regimens was significantly improved in the experimental groups but the difference in relapse rates was only partly accounted for by better compliance.

The use of neuroleptic medication is not just a transaction between schizophrenic patient and prescribing doctor. Many other people are involved – nurses, occupational therapists, rehabilitation workers, family carers, hostel wardens, police and the public-at-large. All these viewpoints must be taken into account in the search for the ideal neuroleptic drug.

The Future

The English poet, Samuel Taylor Coleridge (1772–1834) wrote:

> *"If men could learn from history, what lessons it might teach us! But passion and party blind our eyes, and the light which experience gives is a lantern on the stern, which shines only on the waves behind us."*

However, one group of researchers have reviewed the past dispassionately by conducting a remarkable meta-analysis of one hundred years of outcome literature in schizophrenia (Hegarty et al. 1994). Their conclusions make sombre and sobering reading. They analysed 320 studies with 51 800 subjects from 368 cohorts and 311 400 patient-years of follow-up. Only 40% of patients were improved after follow-ups averaging 5.6 years. The broader the criteria the better the outcome. Outcome improved from 1955 onwards reflecting both improved treatment but also loosening of diagnostic criteria. Ominously, in the decade from 1982 onwards the average rate of favourable outcome declined to 36%, again probably secondary to changes in diagnostic fashions.

Manifestly, the neuroleptic drugs have not revolutionized the natural history of schizophrenia although they may have facilitated the management of many patients. The advent of newer treatments, especially clozapine, has not yet had much impact. Only a fraction of eligible patients in most countries have been tried on clozapine. But even if every treatment-resistant patient was treated with clozapine, the overall effects would still stop short of a major revolution. Of course, schizophrenia is such a serious condition that the improvement wrought by clozapine is important but it will never be the ideal neuroleptic. Nor do any other putative neuroleptics in the pipeline promise much more (Meltzer 1995).

Meanwhile, we can make better, by that I mean more rational, use of the currently-available drugs. Mega-doses and polypharmacy should be discouraged (Johnson 1990). Guidelines on plasma concentration monitoring should be refined and tested under real clinical conditions. The particular problems of treating patients in the community should be specifically addressed (e.g. Lader and Tylee 1994), and not adapted hastily from established usage of drugs on the back wards of asylums.

New drug development is still empirical and the importance of the numerous neurotransmitter systems involved in psychiatric mechanisms remain unclear (Reynolds 1992). Debate continues as to whether the dopamine hypothesis has run out of steam but no successor yet carries the same empirical face validity, at least in terms of general psychotic disturbance rather than specific schizophrenic psychopathology. It may be unrealistic to develop one medication effective in all types of schizophrenia and the subgrouping of schizophrenia on a biological rather than a clinical basis is developing rapidly. I suspect, however, that like most of psychopharmacology, the next break-through in the treatment of schizophrenia, perhaps approximately to the ideal, will come from a serendipitous observation by an astute clinician rather than a science-led basic hypothesis. There is still plenty of work for Hanns Hippius and his like!

References

Balant-Gorgia AE, Balant LP, Andreoli A (1993) Pharmacokinetic optimisation of the treatment of psychosis. Clin Pharmacokinet 25:217–236

Bristow MF, Hirsch SR (1993) Pitfalls and problems of the long term use of neuroleptic drugs in schizophrenia. Drug Saf 8:136–148

Buchanan RW, Holstein C, Breier A (1994) The comparative efficacy and long-term effect of clozapine treatment on neuropsychological test performance. Biol Psychiatry 36:717–725

Cassens G, Inglis AK, Appelbaum PS, Gutheil TG (1990) Neuroleptics: effects on neuropsychological function in chronic schizophrenic patients. Schizophr Bull 16:477–499

Csernansky JG, Newcomer JG (1995) Maintenance drug treatment for schizophrenia. In: Bloom FE, Kupfer DJ (eds) Psychopharmacology: the fourth generation of progress. Raven, New York, pp 1267–1275

Davis JM (1985) Maintenance therapy and the natural course of schizophrenia. J Clin Psychiatry 11:18–21

Davis JM, Metalon L, Watanabe MD, Blake L (1994) Depot antipsychotic drugs. Place in therapy. Drugs 47:741–773

De Jesus Mari J, Streiner DL (1994) An overview of family interventions and relapse on schizophrenia: meta-analysis of research findings. Psychol Med 24:565–578

Dubin WR, Waxman H, Weiss DJ et al (1985) Rapid tranquilization: the efficacy of oral concentrate. J Clin Psychiatry 46:475–478
Farde L, Nordstrom A-L, Wiesel F-A (1992) Positron emission tomographic analysis of central D_1 and D_2 dopamine receptor occupancy in patients treated with classical neuroleptics and clozapine. Arch Gen Psychiatry 49:538–544
Goldberg RJ, Dubin WR, Fogel BS (1989) Behavioral emergencies. Assessment and psychopharmacologic management. Clin Neuropharmacol 12:233–248
Gratz S, Simpson GM (1994) Neuroleptic malignant syndrome. CNS Drugs 2:429–439
Hartmann K, Hiob J, Hippius H (1955) Zur vergleichenden Psychopathologie der Schock- und Phenothiazinwirkungen. Fortschr Neurol Psychiatr 23:345–366
Hegarty JD, Baldessarini RJ, Tohen M, Waternaux C, Oepen G (1994) One hundred years of schizophrenia: a meta-analysis of the outcome literature. Am J Psychiatry 151:1409–1416
Hippius H (1989) The history of clozapine. Psychopharmacology 99:S3–S5
Hoge SK, Appelbaum PS, Lawlor T et al (1990) A prospective, multicenter study of patients' refusal of antipsychotic medication. Arch Gen Psychiatry 47:949–956
Johnson DAW (1990) Pharmacological treatment of patients with schizophrenia. Past and present problems and potential future therapy. Drugs 39:481–488
Jusic N, Lader M (1994) Post-mortem antipsychotic drug concentrations and unexplained deaths. Br J Psychiatry 165:787–791
Kane JM (1993) Newer antipsychotic drugs. A review of their pharmacology and therapeutic potential. Drugs 46:585–593
Kane JM, Lieberman JA (1987) Maintenance pharmacotherapy in schizophrenia. In: Meltzer HY (ed) Psychopharmacology: the third generation of progress. The emergence of molecular biology and biological psychiatry. Raven, New York, pp 1103–1109
Kerwin RW (1994) The new atypical antipsychotics. A lack of extrapyramidal side-effects and new routes in schizophrenia research. Br J Psychiatry 164:141–148
Lader M (1992) Clozapine – a summary. Br J Psychiatry 160 Suppl 17:65–66
Lader M (1994) Historical introduction. Acta Psychiatr Scand 89 Suppl 380:6–7
Lader M (1995) What is relapse in schizophrenia? Int Clin Psychopharmacol 9 Suppl 5:5–9
Lader M, Lewander T (eds) (1994) The neuroleptic-induced deficit syndrome. Acta Psychiatr Scand 89 Suppl 380
Lader MH, Tylee A (eds) (1994) Guidelines for the management of schizophrenia. Lundbeck, Milton Keynes
Lingjærde O (1991) Benzodiazepines in the treatment of schizophrenia: an updated survey. Acta Psychiatr Scand 84:453–459
Meltzer HY (1995) Atypical antipsychotic drugs. In: Bloom FE, Kupfer DJ (eds) Psychopharmacology: the fourth generation of progress. Raven, New York, pp 1277–1286
Newcomer JW, Faustman WO, Yeh W, Czernansky JG (1990) Distinguishing depression and negative symptoms in unmedicated patients with schizophrenia. Psychiatry Res 31:243–250
Nutt DJ (1990) Specific anatomy, non-specific drugs: the present state of schizophrenia. J Psychopharmacol 4:171–175
Pilowski LS, Ring H, Shine PJ, Battersby M, Lader M (1992) Rapid tranquillisation. A survey of emergency prescribing in a general psychiatric hospital. Br J Psychiatry 160:831–835
Prosser ES, Csernansky JG, Kaplan J, Thiemann S, Becker TJ, Hollister LE (1987) Depression, parkinsonian symptoms, and negative symptoms in schizophrenics treated with neuroleptics. J Nerv Ment Dis 175:100–105
Regier DA, Farmer ME, Rae DS et al. (1990) Comorbidity of mental disorders with alcohol and other drugs of abuse: results from the Epidemiologic Catchment Area (ECA) Study. JAMA 264:2511–2518
Reynolds GP (1992) Developments in the drug treatment of schizophrenia. IJPS 131:116–121
Shepherd M (1994) Neurolepsis and the psychopharmacological revolution: myth and reality. History Psychiatry 5:89–96
Smith J, Hucker S (1994) Schizophrenia and substance abuse. Br J Psychiatry 165:13–21
Task Force Report (1987) Sudden death in psychiatric patients: the role of neuroleptic drugs. APA, Washington (American Psychiatric Association report no 27)
Van Putten T (1974) Why do schizophrenic patients refuse to take their drugs? Arch Gen Psychiatry 31:67–72
Van Putten T, Marder SR, Mintz J, Poland RE (1992) Haloperidol plasma levels and clinical response: a therapeutic window relationship. Am J Psychiatry 49:500–505
Volavka J, Cooper T, Czobor P et al (1992) Haloperidol blood levels and clinical effects. Arch Gen Psychiatry 49:354–361

Windgassen K (1992) Treatment with neuroleptics: the patient's perspective. Acta Psychiatr Scand 86:405–410
Wirshing WC, Marder SR, Van Putten T, Arnes D (1995) Acute treatment of schizophrenia. In: Bloom FE, Kupfer DJ (eds) Psychopharmacology: the fourth generation of progress. Raven, New York, pp 1259–1266

Long-Term Treatment of Schizophrenia

J. M. Kane

Introduction

Enormous progress has taken place in several fields from genetics to brain imaging which have advanced knowledge regarding those biologic variables which may play a role in schizophrenia. Tremendous effort has focused on the further understanding of neuropharmacologic mechanisms of action of antipsychotic drugs. These efforts have progressed along two lines, first directed towards developing more effective and or more specific, less toxic treatments for psychotic disorders and second, to test specific hypothesis with regard to mechanism(s) of drug action. These lines of investigation have drawn primarily on knowledge of different neurotransmitter receptors and receptor subtypes. This overview is intended to summarize the current status of long-term antipsychotic drug therapy in the treatment of schizophrenia.

Rationale for Maintenance Treatment

Numerous controlled trials (Davis 1975; Kane and Lieberman 1987) have demonstrated the value of maintenance medication in preventing relapse and rehospitalization. Most recently, Gilbert et al. (1995) reviewed 66 studies on antipsychotic (neuroleptic) withdrawal involving a total of 4365 patients with schizophrenia. The mean cumulative relapse rate across these studies was 53% in patients withdrawn from antipsychotic drugs and 16% in those maintained on medication, over a mean follow-up period of 9.7 months. Despite a number of important differences in the methodology employed in these studies, ranging from diagnostic criteria to definition of relapse, etc., the results are fairly consistent. Those patients who were withdrawn from antipsychotic drugs had a relapse rate which was more than three times higher than the rate of those who were maintained on medication. Baldessarini and Viguera (1995) in their own reanalysis of some of these data pointed out that this difference reaches almost sixfold if the mean ratio of relapse risk within pairs is considered and weighted by the number of subjects in each study.

Although many attempts have been made to identify useful predictors of relapse, the results of these efforts are not consistent nor do they account for a sizable enough proportion of the variance to be meaningful in clinical practice. Those predictors which have been found in some studies to be associated with higher rates of relapse include: earlier age of onset of illness; younger age at time of study; higher doses of neuroleptic medication prior to drug withdrawal; and recency of hospitalization.

In the review by Gilbert et al. (1995), the only specific predictor for relapse was the average length of the follow-up interval – the longer the follow-up the higher the rate of relapse. It is also clear in the studies that they reviewed, however, that a large proportion of the relapse risk occurs early following drug withdrawal. A question remains in many of these reports as to how stable the patients were at the time of drug withdrawal. Given the fact that many of these studies were done in the days when patients were maintained for lengthy periods in hospital, it is unclear whether the results are fully generalizable to discussions of outpatients in relative remission or at a stable clinical plateau. Baldessarini and Viguera (1995) point out that the relative risk between drug discontinuation and maintenance treatment falls over time from 12.9 in the first 3 months to 1.9 at 18 – 24 months.

In general the vast majority of the data available support the enormous value of maintenance medication. The potential risks associated with psychotic relapse and re-hospitalization include: personal suffering; loss of psychosocial and vocational status ; interference with family relationships or housing availability; vulnerability to substance abuse; violent or criminal behavior; aggressive acts and suicide. It is also clear, however, that perhaps as many as half of those patients withdrawn from antipsychotic drugs do not relapse within a period of 6 – 12 months. In view of the potential risk of tardive dyskinesia, this can create a clinical dilemma. We have reported data (Kane, 1995) from a large-scale epidemiologic study suggesting a cumulative incidencs of tardive dyskinesia of approximately 5% per year of antipsychotic drug exposure – at least for the first 8 years of drug treatment. Though the vast majority of these cases are mild and not progressive, this remains a substantial risk. In those patients who are older and particularly those over the age of 50 – 60 the risk is substantially higher, perhaps as great as sixfold (Saltz et al. 1991; Jeste and Calaguri 1993). Because of the risk of tardive dyskinesia and other adverse effects, considerable attention has been focused on issues of dosage and alternative maintenance medication strategies.

Indications for Long-Term Treatment

It is generally agreed upon among most clinical experts that some form of maintenance treatment or relapse prevention is indicated in any patient with a clear diagnosis of schizophrenia (Kissling 1991). In an individual who has had only one schizophrenic or schizophreniform episode, maintenance treatment should be continued for at least 1 and probably 2 years. If a clinical decision is made to discontinue medication at that point, it should probably be done in the context of a targeted or intermittent treatment strategy (to be discussed in detail subsequently) as opposed to leaving the patient without adequate follow-up and without emphasizing the need to be sensitive to the likelihood of a subsequent episode. In the cases of those individuals who have had more than one or two episodes, maintenance treatment should be continued for at least five years and probably indefinitely. Fortunately there are few if any absolute contraindications to prolonged treatment with antipsychotic drugs. Even if tardive dyskinesia does develop, the potential benefits of continued treatment are likely to outweigh the risks.

At the same time there continue to be frequent problems with long-term antipsychotic drug treatment. First, many patients do not respond sufficiently to the acute treatment to be considered recovered or in remission from acute psychosis. For those patients, the goals of maintenance drug therapy are more limited than they are among more responsive patients. Second, even among those individuals who respond very well to medication, residual signs and symptoms may be apparent, particularly varying degrees of negative symptoms, such as diminished drive or motivation and reduced pleasure capacity, blunted affect and lack of spontaneity. Third, antipsychotic drugs are associated with a number of adverse affects which can be subjectively uncomfortable, distressing and even embarrassing or stigmatizing. This is particularly true of the neurologic side effects such as drug-induced parkinsonism, tardive dyskinesia or tardive dystonia. Indeed some of these side effects (i. e., akinesia) may in fact mimic or potentially exacerbate preexisting negative symptoms such as blunted affect, diminish spontaneity, anhedonia or motor retardation. Akathisia on the other hand can mimic anxiety, tension or agitation. Noncompliance in medication-taking continues to be an enormous problem and is one of the most frequent causes of rehospitalization. Although there is a number of causes that can contribute to noncompliance, the occurrence of adverse affects is undoubtedly one of the major determinants.

Dosing in Long-Term Treatment

Prior to any discussion of drug dosage in the maintenance stage of treatment, it is necessary to briefly discuss issues of dosing in the acute treatment phase. It is quite probable that the dosage which a patient receives during the treatment of a relapse or an acute exacerbation will have a substantial influence on the initial maintenance dose. Many patients continue to receive higher than necessary dosages during acute treatment, particularly if they have shown evidence of violent or aggressive behavior (Remington et al. 1993) or have been poor or partial responders to the initial treatment (Quitkin et al. 1975). There is little if any evidence that high doses or "mega" dose treatment is either more effective or more rapid in onset of therapeutic activity than moderate dosages such as haloperidol 20 mg/day or chlorpromazine 600 mg/day. Recent clinical trials support this conclusion in that there is little to be gained by substantial dose increase in comparison to waiting or switching to a different class of antipsychotic drug (Kinon et al. 1993; Shalev et al. 1993).

Although there has not been a clearcut relationship established between dosage requirements for the acute treatment of a psychotic relapse and those dosages required for the prevention of relapse in the maintenance phase of treatment, there has been some suggestion that the dose of antipsychotic drug prior to discontinuing medication may bear some relationship to relapse risk (Prien and Cole 1968; Gilbert et al. 1995). It is likely that dosing levels covary with illness severity and this could explain such a relationship, but it is also possible that rapid withdrawal from a relatively high dose of medication might increase the likelihood of an illness exacerbation or reemergence due to a pharmacodynamic effect. This would argue for a gradual rather than rapid reduction from a relatively high dose during the acute treatment phase to a more modest or low dose in the maintenance treatment phase.

Smith (1994) studied a strategy of very slow dosage reduction in 16 chronically psychotic schizophrenic or schizoaffective patients who had been continuously hospitalized for a mean of 11.5 years. The medication dosage was reduced by one-fifth to one-third of the current dose every 1–2 months, as long as there was no significant clinical exacerbation. A reduction in mean antipsychotic drug dosage of about 60% was achieved over an average follow-up interval of ten months with some actual improvement in measures of psychopathology. A study by Green et al. (1992) suggested that slow antipsychotic drug withdrawal (utilizing a 2-month time frame) was preferable to a more rapid (2-week) withdrawal, in that the latter group experienced a 50% relapse rate over 6 months of follow-up as compared to an 8% relapse rate among those undergoing the more gradual drug withdrawal.

These findings might also suggest a potential advantage for long-acting injectable (depot) drugs in that dosage reduction and ultimately drug withdrawal is a very gradual process due to the pharmacokinetics of these compounds. Baldessarini and Viguera (1995) reported that the mean time to 50% risk for recurrence of illness was 4 months after discontinuance of oral antipsychotics, whereas the 50% risk was not reached until 6.7 months after stopping treatment with depot drugs. This should not be surprising in view of the pharmacokinetics of depot drugs, however, these authors also found that the relapse risk following the discontinuation of depot medications remained lower than that after discontinuing oral medication into the second year (60%–65% versus 85%–90%) raising the possibility that a very slow elimination of medication may in fact reduce the risk of relapse rather than just delaying it.

Attempts in recent years to establish minimum effective dosage requirements for the long-term treatment of schizophrenia have focused on two different approaches. First, the comparison of different fixed dosages of medication in double-blind, random assignment trials and second the comparison of continuous drug treatment with an "intermittent" or "targeted" maintenance strategy. In comparing the outcomes of these studies, it is important to recognize that the methodology employed may have differed somewhat in definitions of relapse, selection criteria, length of trial, etc., yet there is considerable consistency in the results across many of these investigations.

Low-Dose Studies

Continuous low dose medication has been studied in four large-scale clinical trials involving outpatients followed for at least one year. Kane et al. (1983, 1985) studied 163 patients randomly assigned to three different dosage ranges of fluphenazine decanoate: 1.25–5.0 mg, 2.5–10.0 mg, or 12.5–50 mg given every second week. At the end of 1 year the cumulative relapse rates, defined by changes in psychosis on the Brief Psychiatric Rating Scale (BPRS) were 56% on the lowest dose, 24% on the intermediate dose, and 14% on the highest dose. Although there were significant differences in relapse rates, few patients in the lowest dosage range had to be rehospitalized, and on average, those patients who did relapse had returned to their baseline state within nine weeks of having their dosage increased (in response to the relapse). In addition, those individuals who were receiving the lowest dosage also achieved better ratings on some measures of psychosocial adjustment as well as the BPRS items: emotional withdrawal, tension, blunted affect and psychomotor retardation. The fact that some of these differences were apparent to family members who rated the patients on measures of social adjustment suggests that they were not trivial (Kreisman et al. 1988). Although several of these signs are associated with "negative" symptoms, it would appear that their improvement in this dosage reduction paradigm was in all likelihood due to a reduction in extrapyramidal side effects, and they could, therefore, be considered "secondary" negative symptoms.

Marder et al. (1984, 1987) studied 66 male outpatients in a Veterans Affairs Clinic who were randomly assigned to 5 or 25 mg of fluphenazine decanoate given every second week and followed for 2 years. These researchers defined three levels of potential outcome: psychotic exacerbation, relapse, and rehospitalization. A psychotic exacerbation was defined as an increase of three or more points on the BPRS cluster scores for either thought disturbance or paranoia. A relapse was considered to have occurred if patients could not be returned to their baseline state by an increase (of up to 100%) in the dosage that they were receiving. Following an exacerbation, the treating physicians were allowed to increase the dose up to 10 mg for those patients receiving 5 mg, and up to 50 mg for those patients in the 25-mg group. At the end of one year, the exacerbation rates were 35% on 5 mg and 43% on 25 mg, whereas the relapse rates were 22% versus 20%. These differences were nonsignificant. After 2 years of follow-up, however, the two dosages did result in different rates of exacerbation, 69% on the 5 mg dose as compared to 36% on the 25 mg dosage. In terms of relapse rates, the difference remained non-significant (44% on 5 mg and 31% on 25 mg). These results serve to emphasize the importance of a long-term perspective in assessing the impact of maintenance treatment strategies; however, few studies to date have lasted more than 1 year.

Johnson et al. (1987) included 59 stable outpatients in a maintenance treatment study. These individuals had been receiving flupenthixol decanoate up to 40 mg every 2 weeks for at least 1 year. Patients were randomly assigned to either continue their original dose or undergo a 50% dosage reduction. All participating patients were followed for 1 year. A significantly higher relapse rate (32%) was seen in the dose reduction group in comparison to the control patients (10%). After the first year of the study those patients who had originally been assigned to their regular dose had their dose then reduced by 50%, and all patients were followed for an additional 2 years. Of those patients followed on the reduced dose for 3 years 70% experienced a relapse and of those followed on reduced dose for 2 years 56% relapsed. Three out of every four patients had resumed their previous full dose by the end of the follow-up. The full dosage employed here is approximately equivalent to 25 mg of fluphenazine decanoate given every second week. Although there were fewer extrapyramidal side effects experienced by the patients during the low dose treatment, the differences were not statistically significant.

Hogarty et al. (1988) studied 70 stable outpatients who were categorized as living in high expressed emotion (EE) or low EE households. Participants were randomly assigned double-blind to receive a standard dose of fluphenazine decanoate (the mean was 25 mg every 2 weeks) or a minimal dose, approximately 20% of the original dose (mean 3.8 mg every 2 weeks). At the end of 1 year, the relapse rate for those patients receiving the higher dose was 14% as compared to 20% for those in the lower dose group. After 2 years the rates were 24% and 30%, respectively. No significant differences in relapse rates were found between the doses at either 1 or 2 years. Differences in extrapyramidal side effects were significant in favor of the low dose group after the first year, but these differences were not significant after 2 years. These investigators also reported that the lowest dose demonstrated some advantage in terms of being associated with less emotional withdrawal and psychomotor retardation as well as better psychosocial and vocational adjustment as previous reported by Kane (1985).

Kane et al. (1995) have reported data on 105 stable outpatients randomly assigned to one of four different fixed doses of haloperidol decanoate: 200, 100, 50 mg, or 25 mg monthly. Utilizing a priori changes on the psychotic items of the Brief Psychiatric Rating Scale as indicators of clinically significant exacerbation or relapse, these investigators found a 16% relapse rate in the 200-mg group, a 23% relapse rate in the 100-mg group, a 25% relapse rate in the 50-mg group and a relapse rate of 60% in the group receiving 25 mg. The differences among the 50, 100, and 200 mg relapse rates were not statistically significant. It would appear that a substantial proportion of patients can be maintained on doses of haloperidol decanoate between 50 and 100 mg given once per month. Interestingly, the 200 mg per month group did not experience significantly more adverse effects than those patients receiving lower doses.

Taken together the results of these studies suggest that substantial dose reduction is feasible for many patients, though the risk of relapse does increase. The proportion relapsing will increase the lower the dose utilized and the longer the patients are followed. In addition, the less stable the patients are initially, the greater the risk may be. Dose reduction can lead to some diminution in adverse effects, particularly subtle extrapyramidal side effects, though the reduction in risk for the occurrence of tardive dyskinesia is neither consistent nor dramatic. It may be, however, that a relatively brief time frame in the development of tardive dyskinesia (1–2 years) is inadequate to fully determine the impact of these strategies on the long-term incidence of tardive dyskinesia. It might be particularly useful to identify patients at high risk for the development of tardive dyskinesia and then test the impact of specific dosage reduction strategies.

Targeted or Intermittent Medication

Given the fact that many patients do not relapse for several months following the complete discontinuation of antipsychotic medication, a strategy evolved which included complete drug discontinuation, but also intensive follow-up in order to identify the earliest signs of symptom exacerbation or relapse which would then precipitate the reinstitution of medication. The goals of this strategy are therefore somewhat similar to those of the continuous low-dose strategy in the sense of attempting to reduce the risk of tardive dyskinesia, to lessen other side effects, and, therefore, improve subjective well-being, compliance and possibly psychosocial and vocational adjustment. In order to implement this strategy clinicians, patients and their families must be educated to recognize that the prodromal symptoms and exacerbation are highly likely to occur at some point in time and that everyone must collaborate to ensure as rapid intervention as possible with medication in order to prevent or control a further worsening of the patient's condition. Although this same requirement is in effect to some extent in the use of the "low-dose" strategy, in that context the dosage is increased and the patient already has some medication in his/her system.

Another rationale supporting the feasibility of the targeted strategy grew out of the observations of Herz and Melville (1980) that some patients have characteristic prodromal periods with specific signs and symptoms that precede a psychotic episode. They observed that patients and families can frequently recall such early signs of decompensation (e.g., sleep disturbance, irritability, changes in energy level or attention, depression or mild psychotic signs and symptoms).

As Carpenter and Heinrich (1983) have emphasized, this is not a "no medication" strategy, but it is rather an alternative approach to using medication in the context of long-term management.

Four large scale studies have been published involving targeted or intermittent treatment. Herz et al. (1991) completed a double-blind study in 140 subjects. Intermittently treated patients did receive significantly less medication; however, they were also significantly less likely to complete the 2-year study course (38% versus 72%). Patients receiving continuous medication went for significantly longer periods of time without prodromal episodes or full relapses.

Carpenter et al. (1990) published a study involving 116 newly discharged patients. Treatment was not blind. Targeted patients received medication only 52% of the time; however, significantly more patients in the continuous-treatment group completed the full two year study. Patients on targeted treatment experienced significantly more clinical exacerbations and were more likely to be hospitalized. For those patients who were still in treatment after the 2 years, the degree of job employment was significantly better among those receiving continuous medication.

A group of British investigators (Hirsh et al. 1987; Jolley et al. 1989, 1990) reported on 54 outpatients with schizophrenia who were randomly assigned, double-blind to continuous or intermittent treatment. These investigators reported no significant differences in the number of patients completing the first year of the trial in each group, however, significantly more patients receiving the intermittent treatment (76%) experienced prodromal episodes as compared to those in the continuous-treatment group (27%). In addition, the intermittent group experienced significantly more relapses, but the number of hospitalizations did not differ. In the second year of the trial, although the intermittently treated group continued to receive less medication overall, both the rates of relapse and rehospitalization were significantly greater in the intermittent group. Although there had been a trend toward a lower incidence of tardive dyskinesia observed at the end of the first year in this study, this was not seen at the end of two years.

Pietzcker et al. (1986) have conducted a trial comparing standard maintenance medication, neuroleptic crisis intervention, and prophylactic early neuroleptic intervention. The investigators studied 365 patients at four different sites. The neuroleptic crisis intervention group included in this study differs from the intermittent treatment concept in that this group received medication only when a relapse occurred rather than at the identification of early or prodromal symptoms. This study, therefore, provided an opportunity to assess whether or not intervention at the prodromal symptom phase could prevent the development of a full blown relapse. At both 1 and 2 years, patients in the early intervention group experienced a significantly higher relapse rate compared to the standard maintenance treatment group. The rate of rehospitalization was not significantly greater in the first year (23% versus 16%), but did reach significance in the second year (37% versus 24%). Those patients receiving only the crisis intervention with neuroleptic drugs had a significantly higher relapse rate than the other two groups.

Although there are a number of differences in design and methodology among the studies, there is considerable agreement in terms of results. It would appear that an intermittent treatment strategy is feasible and can be implemented in ambulatory care settings. In addition, this approach can result in reduced cumulative neuroleptic exposure and, to some extent, a reduction in adverse effects. However, the disadvantages include an increase in the risk of prodromal episodes, relapse and rehospitalization. It is particularly disappointing to recognize that no consistent benefits of intermittent treatment have been demonstrated in terms of improving psychosocial or vocational functioning or reducing the risk of tardive dyskinesia. Some patients may be particularly poor candidates for this approach because their relapses are associated with severe loss of insight, risk of suicidal behavior or a history of aggressiveness or assaultiveness.

On the other hand, those patients who absolutely refuse to comply with continuous medication, but who with proper education and psychosocial support might comply with an intermittent strategy, could be considered appropriate candidates. In addition, with patients who have only had one psychotic episode and for whom there is a consensus that a trial off of medication may be justifiable, the intermittent or targeted strategy should be the approach that is taken.

It has also been suggested from a handful of studies that intermittent treatment rather than reducing the potential risk of tardive dyskinesia may in fact increase it (Jeste et al. 1979; Kane 1995; Goldman and Luchins 1984).

Depot Medication

It is important to note that almost all of the studies involving comparisons of different dosages in the long-term treatment of schizophrenia have employed depot medication. Investigators conducting these clinical trials needed to be certain that patients in fact received the amount of medication intended, otherwise it would be very difficult to make potentially subtle distinctions between the benefit-to-risk ratios of specific dosing strategies. When patients are treated with oral medication, it is often difficult to ascertain the level of compliance. A relapse may be precipitated by noncompliance or noncompliance may be a secondary effect of the early stages of a relapse. Among patients receiving long-acting injectable medications, it is obvious if and when a patient has missed an injection and is therefore not receiving the prescribed medication. It is also apparent that there is less interindividual variability in the relationship between dosage administered and blood level achieved when medication is given parenterally (Nayak et al. 1987). Intramuscular injections increase bioavailability and reduce the first-pass hepatic effect. Studies have demonstrated a better correlation between dosage and blood levels when medications are administered by injection (Davis et al. 1994). Once dosage guidelines are established, therefore, giving medication via a depot drug allows the clinician greater control over dosage and confidence as to whether or not the desired level of pharmacotherapy is being achieved.

Clearly, the most important advantage of depot antipsychotic medications is in reducing the risk of noncompliance. Noncompliance in medicationtaking occurs in probably 30%–50% of patients over a 1-year period (Kane 1986; Mann 1986). Six double-blind, random-assignment prospective studies (del Guidice et al. 1975; Rifkin et al. 1977; Hogarty et al. 1979; Schooler et al. 1980; Falloon et al. 1978; Crawford and Forrest 1974) have been conducted comparing relapse rates of patients on oral and depot medication. Although the average difference in relapse between the two treatments was 15%, favoring depot drugs, when the data from these studies were combined utilizing the Mantel-Haenszel test (Mantel and Haenszel 1959) a highly significant difference ($\chi^2 = 13.5$, $p = .0002$) was evident favouring depot drugs (Davis et al. 1989).

We have argued (Kane and Borenstein 1985) that these results probably underestimate the true impact of depot medications, because those patients who were studied had to be cooperative and compliant enough to be willing to participate in a controlled clinical trial. In such trials patients are monitored closely, seen more frequently and assessed more carefully which may also enhance compliance. In all likelihood for many patients noncompliance is a gradually developing phenomenon and when it does result in the complete discontinuation of medication the consequences (in terms of relapse) are not seen immediately, but usually occur after an average of 3–7 months. It is not surprising, therefore, that in the study by Hogarty et al. (1979) which was the only one that lasted more than 1 year, relapse rates were much higher in the second year on oral medication as compared to depot therapy.

In the general population of patients with schizophrenia, it is fairly safe to assume that more widespread use of depot drugs could substantially reduce rates of relapse and rehospitalization thereby decreasing personal suffering, family burden and social costs. The reasons why these agents are infrequently used in many settings are not always clear. It is probable that some clinicians are unduly concemed about adverse effects and/or patient acceptance of depot injections.

Reviews of the literature (Glazer and Kane 1992) do not support any greater risk of adverse effects associated with depot drugs when comparisons are made with equivalent doses of oral medication. In terms of patient acceptance, it is often the clinicians themselves who have a bias against depot drugs which they frequently view as too intrusive or controlling and not encouraging of patient autonomy. In addition, they often associate depot drugs with the highly uncooperative patients. In reality our experience suggests that the vast majority of patients will accept depot medication if the clinician patiently discusses the pros and cons over a period of time; and, in fact, many patients prefer regular injections over having to take oral medication on a daily basis (Diamond 1983).

Conclusion

Major progress has been made in recent years in further establishing the benefits and risks of maintenance treatment. In addition, a substantial amount of new knowledge is available regarding alternative dosing strategies. This is especially true for long-acting injectable medication. There is no question that long-term treatment with antipsychotic drugs is a cornerstone of successful treatment. At the same time, however, appropriate attention to issues of dosage, adverse effects, compliance, as well as psychosocial treatment strategies and psychoeducation for both patients and families is necessary to maximize the potential for the best possible outcome.

References

Baldessarini RJ, Viguera AC (1995) Neuroleptic withdrawal in schizophrenic patients. Arch Gen Psychiatry 52:189–192

Carpenter WT Jr, Heinrichs D (1983) Early intervention, time limited, targeted pharmacothrapy of schizophrenia. Schizophr Bull 9:533–542

Carpenter WT Jr, Hanlon TE, Heinrichs DW, Kirkpatrick B, Levine J, Buchanan RW (1990) Continuous vs. targeted medication in schizophrenic outpatients: outcome results. Am J Psychiatry 147:1138–1148

Crawford R, Forrest A (1974) Controlled trial of depot fluphenazine in outpatient schizophrenics. Br J Psychiatry 124: 385–391

Davis JM (1975) Overview: maintenance therapy in psychiatry. I. Schizophrenia. Am J Psychiatry 132:1237–1245

Davis JM, Barter JT, Kane JM (1989) Antisychotic drugs. In: Kaplan HA, Sadock (eds) Comprehensive textbook of psychiatry, 5th edn. Williams and Wilkins, Baltimore, pp 1591–1626

Davis JM, Metalon L, Watanabe MD, Blake L (1994) Depot antipsychotic drugs – place in therapy. Drugs 47(5):741–773

Diamond RJ (1983) Enhancing medication use in schizophrenic patients. J Clin Psychiatry 44:7–14

Falloon I, Watt DC, Shepherd M (1978) A comparative controlled trial of pimozide and fluphenazine decanoate in the continuation therapy of schizophrenia. Psychol Med 8:59–70

Gilbert PL, Harris MJ, McAdams LA, Jeste DV (1995) Neuroleptic withdrawal in schizophrenic patients: a review of the literature. Arch Gen Psychiatry 52:173–188

del Giudice J, Clark WG, Gocka EF (1975) Prevention of recidivism of schizophrenics treated with fluphenazine enanthate. Psychosomatics 16:32–36

Glazer WM, Kane JM (1992) Depot neuroleptic therapy: an underutilized treatment option. J Clin Psychiatry 53:426–433

Goldman MB, Luchins DJ (1984) Intermittent neuroleptic therapy and tardive dyskinesia. A literature review. Hosp Community Psychiatry 35:1215–1219

Green AI (1992) Neuroleptic dose reduction studies: clinical and neuroendocrine effects. Presented at the 31st Annual Meeting, American College of Neuropsychopharmacology, 14–18 December, San Juan, Puerto Rico

Herz MI, Melville C (1980) Relapse in Schizophrenia. Am J Psychiatry 137 (7): 801–805

Herz MI, Glazer WM, Mostert MA et al (1991) Intermittent vs. maintenance medication in schizophrenia: two-year results. Arch Gen Psychiatry 48:333–339

Hirsch SR, Jolley AG, Manchanda R, McRink A (1987) Early intervention medication as an alternative to continuous depot treatment in schizophrenia: preliminary report. In: Strauss J, Boker W, Brenner HD (eds) Psychosocial treatment of schizophrenia. Huber, Bern, pp 63–72

Hogarty GE, Schooler NR, Ulrich R et al (1979) Fluphenazine and social therapy in the aftercare of schizophrenic patients: relapse analyses of a two-year controlled study of fluphenazine decanoate and fluphenazine hydrochloride. Arch Gen Psychiatry 36: 1283–1294

Hogarty GE, McEvoy JP, Munetz M, DiBarry AL et al (1988) Dose of fluphenazine, familial expressed emotion, and outcome in schizophrenia. Arch Gen Psychiatry 45: 797–805
Jeste DV, Caliguiri MP (1993) Tardive dyskinesia. Schizophr Bull 19:303–315
Jeste DV, Potkin SG, Sinha S, Feder SL, Wyatt RJ (1979) Tardive dyskinesia: reversible and persistent. Arch Gen Psychiatry 36:585–590
Johnson DAW, Ludlow JM, Street K, Taylor RDW (1987) Double-blind comparison of half-dose and standard flupenthixol decanoate in the maintenance treatment of stabilized outpatients with schizophrenia. Br J Psychiatry 151:634–638
Jolley AG, Hirsch SR, McRink A, Manchanda R (1989) Trial of brief intermittent prophylaxis for selected schizophrenia outpatients: clinical outcome at one year. BMJ 298:985–990
Jolley AG, Hirsh SR, Morrison E, McRink A, Wilson L (1990) Trial of brief intermittent prophylaxis for selected schizophrenic outpatients: clinical and social outcome at two years. BMJ 301:837–842
Kane JM (1986) Prevention and treatment of neuroleptic noncompliance. Psychiatr Ann 16:576–578
Kane JM (1995) Tardive dyskinesia. Presentation at the International Congress on Schizophrenia Research. Warm Springs, Virginia, 10–13 April
Kane JM, Borenstein M (1985) Compliance in the long-term treatment of schizophrenia. Psychopharmacol Bull 21:23–27
Kane JM, Lieberman JA (1987) Maintenance pharmacotherapy in schizophrenia. In: Meltzer HY (ed) Psychopharmacology: the third generation of progress. Raven, New York, pp 1103–1109
Kane JM, Rifkin A, Woerner MG, Reardon GT, Sarantakos S, Schiebel D, Ramos-Lorenzi J (1983) Low-dose neuroleptic treatment of outpatient schizophrenics. Arch Gen Psychiatry 40:893–896
Kane JM, Rifkin A, Woerner MG, Reardon GT, Kreisman D, Blumenthal R, Borenstein M (1985) High-dose versus low-dose strategies in the treatment of schizophrenia. Psychopharmacol Bull 21:533–537
Kane JM, Davis JM, Schooler N, Marder S, Casey D, Brauzer B (1995) A multi-dose study of haloperidol decanoate in the maintenance treatment of schizophrenia. Arch Gen Psychiatry (submitted)
Kinon BJ, Kane JM, Johns C, Perovich R, Ismi M, Koreen A, Weiden P (1993) Treatment of neuroleptic-resistant schizophrenic relapse. Psychopharmacol Bull 29:309–314
Kissling W (1991) Guidelines for neuroleptic relapse prevention in schizophrenia. Springer, Berlin Heidelberg New York
Kreisman D, Blumenthal R, Borenstein M et al. (1988) Family attitudes and patient social adjustment in a longtudinal study of outpatient schizophrenics receiving low-dose neuroleptics: the family's view. Psychiatry 51:3–13
Mann JJ (1986) How medication compliance effects outcome. Psychiatr Ann 16:567–570
Mantel N, Haenszel W (1959) Statistical aspects of the analysis of data from retrospective studies of disease. J Natl Cancer Inst 22:719–748
Marder SR, Van Putten T, Mintz J, McKenzie J, Lebell M, Faltico G, May PRA (1984) Costs and benefits of two doses of fluphenazine. Arch Gen Psychiatry 41:1025–1029
Marder SR, Van Putten T, Mintz J, Lebell M, McKenzie J, May PRA (1987) Low and conventional dose maintenance therapy with fluphenazine decanoate: two-year outcome. Arch Gen Psychiatry 44:510–517
Nayak RK, Doose DR, Nair NPV (1987) The bioavailability and pharmacokinetics of oral and depot intramuscular haloperidol in schizophrenia patients. J Clin Pharmacol 27(2): 144–150
Pietzcker A, Gaebel W, Kopcke W, Linden M et al (1986) A German multicenter study on the neuroleptic long-term therapy of schizophrenic patients: preliminary report. Pharmacopsychiatry 19:161–166
Prien RF, Cole JO (1968) High dose of chlorpromazine in chronic schizophrenia. Arch Gen Psychiatry 18:482–495
Quitkin F, Rifkin A, Klein DF (1975) Very high dosage versus standard dosage fluphenazine in schizophrenia. A double-blind study of non-chronic treatment refractory patients. Arch Gen Psychiatry 32:1276–1281
Remington G, Pollock B, Voineskos G, Reed K, Coulter K (1993) Acutely psychotic patients receiving high-dose haloperidol therapy. J Clin Psychopharmacol 13:41–45
Rifkin A, Quitkin F, Rabiner CJ et al (1977) Fluphenazine decanoate, fluphenazine hydrochloride given orally, and placebo in remitted schizophrenics. I. Relapse rates after one year. Arch Gen Psychiatry 34:43–47

Saltz BL, Woerner MG, Kane JM et al (1991) Prospective study of tardive dyskinesia incidence in the elderly. JAMA 266:2402–2406
Schooler NR, Levine J, Severe JB et al. (1980) Prevention of relapse in schizophrenia: an evaluation of fluphenazine decanoate. Arch Gen Psychiatry 37:16–24
Shalev A, Hermesh H, Rothberg J, Munitz H (1993) Poor neuroleptic response in acutely exacerbated schizophrenic patients. Acta Psychiatr Scand 87:86–91
Smith RC (1994) Lower-dose therapy with traditional neuroleptics in chronically hospitalized schizophrenic patients. Arch Gen Psychiatry 51:427–429

Treatment of Affective Disorders

S. A. Montgomery

Recent years have seen considerable improvements in the treatment of depression. Advances have taken place in several directions which include the introduction of improved antidepressants, the general acceptance of the illness as a chronic disorder that is recurrent in the majority of cases and increased knowledge about differential response to treatment in different forms of depression.

The Need for New Antidepressant Treatments

The impetus to develop new antidepressants has been the need for effective treatments that are safer and better tolerated than the traditional tricyclic antidepressants (TCA). When they were introduced the early TCAs represented an important step forward in the approach to managing depression. However, whilst being effective, their usefulness is limited by the unwanted side effects. There is also considerable concern about the safety of the older TCAs, their effect on cardiac function and the associated danger in those with compromised cardiac status and particularly in overdose. Examination of the deaths from poisoning to derive a lethality index in overdose has shown the high risk associated with, for example, amitriptyline and dothiepin compared with other more recently introduced antidepressants (Cassidy and Henry 1987).

The anticholinergic side effects of the TCAs are well known. Patients often find them difficult tolerate and these side effects are frequently cited as the reason for patients discontinuing with treatment. In usual clinical practice at least 60% of patients have been found to stop treatment with TCAs prematurely (Johnson 1981). The difficulty in achieving good compliance with medication contributes to the therapeutic failure of TCAs and is a serious problem as a patient who discontinues treatment because of side effects may well lose confidence in treatment and be lost to care. Because of the side effects, it is common for these antidepressants to be given in very low, often subtherapeutic doses prolonging the illness rather than instituting vigorous treatment. The strategy of starting with low doses and gradually raising the dose is not always successful, as it is sometimes difficult to reach the full therapeutic dose.

The heavy side effect burden of the older TCAs has no doubt contributed to negative perception of antidepressant treatments which discourages sufferers from seeking help. This is unfortunate since depression is a serious illness associated with increased mortality from suicide, increased incidence of physical disease, and a greater level of dysfunction than many common medical conditions (Wells et al. 1989). In spite of the consequences of such a serious condition, only a small proportion of sufferers with depression seek treatment and of those who do, only a small percentage receive adequate treatment (Keller 1988; Keller et al. 1992).

Selective Serotonin Reuptake Inhibitors

The basic concept underlying how antidepressants are thought to work has not changed radically for the development of recent antidepressants, but the recognition that treatments need to be acceptable to patients in order to be effective, has led to the arrival of newer, safer antidepressants lacking the shortcomings of the older compounds. A useful example is provided by the selective serotonin reuptake inhibitors (SSRI) which were developed as antidepressants in response to the need to produce drugs that were more selective in their pharmacological effect in order to avoid the side effects on transmitter systems that do not contribute to the therapeutic response.

This class of drugs has been a considerable success story with efficacy demonstrated compared to placebo and equivalent efficacy to the reference TCAs used as comparators in the large clinical trial programmes (Montgomery 1995). The comparator antidepressants have included imipramine, amitriptyline, clomipramine, maprotiline, as well as oxaprotiline, mianserin and dothiepin, and in general in the direct comparisons no significant differences have been reported. Very large numbers of patients are required to establish equivalent efficacy and the smaller active comparator studies could only provide supporting evidence. Most have reported similar efficacy between the reference and the SSRI with occasional reports of an advantage for the SSRI (Feighner and Boyer 1989; Muijen et al. 1988) or for less efficacy (Andersen et al. 1986). Meta-analyses of the large databases from the clinical trial programmes, which can provide a more reliable estimate of relative efficacy have shown the SSRIs to be of the same order of efficacy as the reference TCAs (Pande and Sayler 1993; Dunbar et al. 1991).

The particular advantage of these newer antidepressants therefore is not that they demonstrate a significant increase in efficacy. Their important advantage lies in their improved side effect profile which makes them better tolerated than the older TCAs. The direct benefit is that patients can be more readily persuaded to persist with treatment at a full therapeutic dose for an adequate course of antidepressants to ensure sustained response. There has been considerable discussion as to whether the cost of newer antidepressants can be justified, when cheap, effective older TCAs are available. Four meta-analyses of the published literature have addressed the relative tolerability of SSRIs compared with TCAs. Three of these included comparisons of TCAs and SSRIs and the fourth, by Song et al. (1993) misleadingly included well-tolerated atypical antidepressants such as mianserin, trazodone and nomifensine among the TCAs. The conclusions of the three straightforward comparisons, which used different methodologies, were in agreement that the SSRIs are of equivalent efficacy, but significantly better tolerated than TCAs with fewer discontinuations due to side effects (Montgomery et al. 1994; Montgomery and Kasper 1995; Anderson and Tomenson 1995).

A drop-out from treatment because of unnecessary side effects is considered to be a real treatment failure. It is difficult enough to persuade patients to take antidepressants without their being discouraged by intolerable side effects.

Particular Antidepressants for Certain Depression

Some interesting evidence of differential effect has been produced in the course of the clinical trial programmes with the newer antidepressants. Most studies are too small to stratify patients into subgroups so that the evidence has come from the larger metanalyses.

Severe Depression

When a new antidepressant is introduced clinicians are eager to know, whether it will be effective in the full range of depression they are likely to encounter.

They are often particularly concerned, if it will be effective in severe depression which is where they may feel least comfortable in prescribing an antidepressant with which they are not familiar. In the meta-analyses of large databases it has been possible to categorise patients into moderate or severe depression on the basis of the severity at entry to the studies and compare the response in the different categories to the new and reference antidepressants. This approach has produced evidence to support the efficacy of the SSRIs in both moderate and severe depression (Montgomery 1989) and in some cases there appears to be a better response to the SSRI in the severe depression group than to the reference TCA (Montgomery 1992; Mendlewicz 1992).

While caution is need in accepting the results from meta-analyses which are beset by methodological difficulties, the finding of improved efficacy in severe depression is important as this is a group where response to a TCA is often poor.

Anxiety in Depression

There is evidence that some antidepressants have a particularly beneficial effect on the anxiety symptoms of depression. Sedative TCAs have traditionally been used to treat depression where the anxiety symptoms are prominent, but it is clear from recent studies that the sedative effect does not carry over into an improvement in the response of the anxiety. In a comparison of amitriptyline and zimelidine the nonsedative SSRI was seen to have a significantly beneficial effect on the anxiety symptoms in depression compared with the sedative TCA (Montgomery et al. 1981). Meta-analyses of the large databases of three SSRIs (fluvoxamine, fluoxetine and paroxetine) have all reported an advantage for the SSRI. The advantage is reflected in an earlier response of the anxiety symptoms measured on the Hamilton Rating Scale for depression (Montgomery 1989; Montgomery 1992; Wakelin 1988).

Nefazadone, a new serotonin reuptake inhibitor with $5HT_2$ antagonist properties appears to have specific advantages in treating the anxiety associated with depression. Nefazadone was seen to reduce the anxiety compared with placebo as early as the first week whereas imipramine, the comparator, appeared to be no different from placebo (Montgomery 1995 b).

Antidepressants and the Risk of Suicide

Depression is associated with a well-known increased risk of suicide and some 15% of individual with major depression eventually commit suicide. It is of considerable concern that antidepressants may provide the undetected suicidal patient with the means with which to harm themselves. Clearly developing safer drugs in overdose, which has been one of the important goals of new antidepressant development, has been of major importance.

There is increasing concern about the high and predictable completed suicide rate with the TCAs. These drugs are thought to be fatal in overdose largely because of their cardiotoxic properties and the deaths from overdose closely parallel the cardiotoxicity seen in animal studies. In a recent analysis (Henry et al. 1995) it was reported that TCAs were associated with around 35 deaths from overdose per million prescriptions in the United Kingdom judged on coroners' death certificates, where death was attributed to the drug on its own. The SSRIs by contrast were associated with a very low level of 2 deaths per million prescriptions. In terms of toxicity in overdose alone the TCAs should not be used as first line treatments. Clinicians would be wise to turn to the newer, safer alternatives rather than using the traditional TCAs with their associated risks.

Suicidal Thoughts in Depressed Patients

Because there are no reliable ways to identify the suicidal patient, it is of considerable interest to clinicians that some antidepressants may be more effective than others in alleviating suicidal thinking. Several of the early studies reported a differential advantage for SSRIs compared with comparator TCAs in their effect on suicidal thoughts (Montgomery et al. 1981; Muijen et al. 1988). Interestingly in the large meta-analysis of the paroxetine database the SSRI was associated with a faster and better reduction of suicidal thoughts compared both with placebo and the comparator antidepressant (Montgomery et al. 1995). A similar advantage is also seen in the analysis of the fluvoxamine database (Wakelin 1988). This suggests that serotonergic drugs have a directly beneficial effect on suicidal thoughts over and above the effect on depression.

Meta-analyses carried out on the large databases from clinical trials also show that the SSRIs exercise a protective effect against the appearance of suicidal thoughts during the course of treatment. Suicidal thoughts are an integral part of depressive illness and fluctuate during the course of an episode as can be seen in the analysis of response to treatment in the meta-analyses of the SSRI databases (Beasley et al. 1991; Montgomery et al. 1995). The databases have been scrutinized for the possibility that the SSRIs might provoke suicidal thoughts by investigating the course of response of patients entering studies with zero or very low scores on suicidal thoughts items of rating scales. These analyses have shown that an increase in suicidal thoughts during treatment is significantly higher on placebo than on active drugs.

The Need for Long-Term Treatment

It is now acknowledged that depression is a long-term illness which recurs in the majority of patients. Studies of the natural history of affective disorders suggest that 15%–20% of patients experience a chronic course and 75%–80% of patients experience recurrent depression (Angst 1992). The recognition of the need for continued treatment to consolidate response and for long-term treatment to prevent new episodes of depression is beginning to inform clinical practice. Much education is still needed both for clinicians and sufferers in order to increase awareness of the benefits of a robust long-term treatment approach to depression.

Adequate Length of Treatment of an Episode of Depression

There is now general agreement that all episodes of major depression require treatment beyond the point at which there is apparent response. It is insufficient to treat an acute episode for the customary 4–6 weeks that is the standard period adopted for testing the efficacy of an antidepressant. The antidepressants appear to ameliorate the symptoms to the point of response but not to cure, and if discontinued early numerous placebo-controlled studies have shown that between 30% and 50% of patients may expect their depressive symptoms to return early in the ensuing months (Mindham et al. 1973; Prien and Kupfer 1986; Montgomery and Dunbar 1993; Montgomery et al. 1993).

The antidepressants that have been recently introduced, have been subjected to more stringent efficacy testing than was the case when the early TCAs were developed and as a result we have a much clearer idea of their therapeutic scope. In Europe is now required that antidepressants should have demonstrated safety and efficacy in long-term treatment since it is accepted that this is how they will be used in practice. The formal placebo-controlled studies have provided incontrovertible evidence of the effectiveness of continuing antidepressant therapy for 4–6 months following response in preventing early relapse. Current programmes for increasing awareness and improving the management of depression are in accord in recommending the need to continue antidepressant treatment for 4–6 months following response in all episodes of depression (Montgomery et al. 1993; WHO Mental Health Collaborating Centres 1995).

In patients with recurrent depression there is good evidence that full doses of antidepressant are required to reduce the risk of new episodes. Imipramine has been rather thoroughly studied and full doses (approximately 200 mg) have been found to be better than placebo and better than psychotherapy (Frank et al. 1990, 1993). There are few data to support the efficacy of other TCAs, but it is likely, if they are used in full therapeutic doses, they may well be effective (reviewed in Montgomery and Montgomery 1992). However one must remember that nortriptyline in a small, but well-designed study, was not found to be effective (Georgotas et al. 1989).

The SSRIs have been well investigated in long-term treatment and paroxetine, sertraline and fluoxetine have all been found to be effective in preventing new episodes of depression in placebo controlled studies (Montgomery et al. 1988; Doogan and Caillard 1992; Montgomery and Dunbar 1993).

Do Placebo Responders Require Antidepressants To Prevent Relapse?

The efficacy of citalopram in preventing relapse following response of the acute episode was tested in a 6-month study in which patients who had responded during a double blind trial of the efficacy of citalopram 40 g or 20 mg compared with placebo were randomized to continuation treatment with placebo or the same dose to which they had responded (Montgomery et al. 1992, 1993). In order to preserve blindness those patients who had responded to placebo in acute treatment were continued double blind on placebo during the continuation treatment study.

In this study there was a significantly higher relapse rate in the patients treated with placebo than with citalopram 40 or 20 mg. The patients who had responded to citalopram were analysed separately and it might have been expected that these patients would remain well. However these patients relapsed at a very similar rate to the patients who had responded to an antidepressant and who were randomized to receive placebo and was significantly higher than patients continued on antidepressant.

This somewhat unexpected finding undermines the general assumption that placebo responders do not require further treatment and has important clinical implications. The response to placebo appears not to have been a true response but a temporary response with substantial risk of relapse. These apparent responders therefore need very careful follow-up in order to institute treatment when relapse occurs.

Conclusion

The improved methodology and the large number of patients included in clinical efficacy trials has enabled us to examine whether certain drugs have particular therapeutic advantages. The TCAs appear to be more dangerous than previously thought and their sedative properties confer no selective advantages in anxious depressions. In contrast SSRIs have been found to have particular therapeutic advantages in treating the anxiety associated with depression in reducing suicidal thoughts faster than TCAs and in treating severe depression. Their major advantage in clinical use however stems from their favourable side effect profile, their comparative safety in overdose, and their significantly improved tolerability compared with the TCAs in ordinary clinical practice.

References

Andersen J, Bech P, Benjaminsen S et al (1986) Citalopram: clinical effect profiles in comparison with clomipramine. A controlled multicentre study. Pschychopharmacology 90:131–138
Anderson IM, Tomenson BM (1995) Treatment discontinuation with selective serotonin reuptake inhibitors compared with tricyclic antidepressants: a meta-analysis. British Medical Journal 310:1433–1438
Angst J (1992) How recurrent and predictable is depressive illness? In: Montgomery SA, Rouillon F (eds) Long-term treatment of depression. Wiley, Chichester, pp 1–14
Beasley CM, Dornseif BE, Bosomworth JC (1991) Fluoxetine and suicidality: absence of association in controlled depression trials. BMJ 303:685–692
Cassidy S, Henry J (1987) Fatal toxicity of antidepressant drugs in overdose. BMJ 295:1021–1024
Doogan DP, Caillard V (1992) Sertraline in the prevention of depression. Br J Psychiatry 160:217–222
Dunbar GC, Cohn JB, Fabre LF, Feighner JP, Fieve RR, Mendels J, Shrivastava RK (1991) A comparison of paroxetine, imipramine and placebo in depressed out-patients. Br J Psychiatry 159:394–398
Feighner JP, Boyer WF (1989) Paroxetine in the treatment of depression: a comparison with imipramine and placebo. Acta Psychiatr Scand 80 [Suppl] 35:125–129
Frank E, Kupfer DJ, Perel JM, Cornes C, Jarrett DB, Mallinger AG, Thase ME, McEachran AB, Grochocinski VJ (1990) Three-year outcomes for maintenance therapies in recurrent depression. Arch Gen Psychiatry 47:1093–1099
Frank E, Kupfer DJ, Perel JM, Cornes C, Mallinger AG, Thase ME, McEachran AB, Grochocinski VJ (1993) Comparison of full-dose versus half-dose pharmacotherapy in the maintenance treatment of recurrent depression. J Affect Disord 27:139–145
Georgotas A, McCue, RE, Cooper TB (1989) A placebo controlled comparison of nortiptyline and phenelzine in maintenance therapy of elderly depressed patients. Arch Gen Psychiatry 46:783–786
Henry JA, Alexander CA, Sener EK (1995) Relative mortality from overdose of antidepressants. BMJ 310:221–224
Johnson DAW (1981) Depression: treatment compliance in general practice. Acta Psychiatr Scand 63 [Suppl 290]:447–453
Keller MB (1988) Undertreatment of major depression. Psychopharmacol Bull 24:75–80
Keller MB, Lavori PW, Mueller TI, Endicott J, Coryell WS, Hirschfeld RMA, Shea MT (1992) Time to recovery, chronicity, and levels of psychopathology in major depression: a 5-year prospective follow-up of 431 subjects. Arch Gen Psychiatry 49:809–816
Mendlewicz J (1992) Efficacy of fluvoxamine in severe depression. Drugs 43 [Suppl 2]:32–39
Mindham RHS, Howland C, Shepherd M (1973) An evaluation of continuation therapy with tricyclic antidepressants in depressive illness. Psychol Med 3:5–17
Montgomery SA, McAulay R, Rani SJ, Roy D, Montgomery DB (1981) A double blind comparison of zimelidine and amitriptyline in endogenous depression. Acta Psychiatr Scand 63 [Suppl 290]:314–327
Montgomery SA, Dufour H, Brion S, Gailledreau J, Lequeille X, Ferrey G, Moron P, Parant-Lucena N, Singer L, Danion JM, Beuzen JN, Pierredoin MA (1988) The prophylactic efficacy of fluoxetine in unipolar depression. Br J Psychiatry 153 [Suppl 3]:69–76
Montgomery SA (1989) The efficacy of fluoxetine as an antidepressant in the short and long term. Int Clin Psychopharmacol 4 [Suppl 1]:113–119
Montgomery SA (1992) The advantages of paroxetine in different subgroups of depression. Inter Clin Psychopharmacol, 6 (S 4), 91–100
Montgomery SA, Montgomery DB (1992) Prophylactic treatment in recurrent unipolar depression. In: Montgomery SA, Rouillon F (eds) Long Term Treatment of Depression. John Wiley & Sons, Chichester, pp 53–80
Montgomery SA, Dunbar GC (1993) Paroxetine is better than placebo in relapse prevention and the prophylaxis of recurrent depression. Int Clin Psychopharmacol 8:189–195
Montgomery SA, Rasmussen JGC, Lyby K, Connor P, Tanghoj P (1992) Dose response relationship of citalopram 20 mg, citalopram 40 mg, and placebo in the treatment of moderate and severe depression. Int Clin Psychopharmacol 6 [Suppl 5]:65–70
Montgomery SA, Bebbington PE, Cowen P, Deakin W, Freeling P, Hallstrom C, Katona C, King D, Leonard B, Levine S, Phanjoo A, Peet M, Thompson C (1993a) Guidelines for treating depressive illness with antidepressants. J Psychopharmacol 7:19–23

Montgomery SA, Rasmussen JGC, Tanghoj P (1993b) A 24 week study of 20 mg citalopram, 40 mg citalopram and placebo in the prevention of relapse of major depression. Int Clin Psychopharmacol 8:181-188
Montgomery SA, Henry J, McDonald G, Dinan T, Lader M, Hindmarch I, Clare A, Nutt D (1994) Selective serotonin reuptake inhibitors: meta-analysis of discontinuation rates. Int Clin Psychpharmacol 9:47-53
Montgomery SA (1995) Selective serotonin reuptake inhibitors in the acute treatment of depression. In: Bloom FE, Kupfer DJ (eds) Psychopharmacology, the fourth generation of progress. Raven, New York, pp 1043-1051
Montgomery SA (1995b) Comparative studies of nefazadone indepression. J. Psychopharmacol (in press)
Montgomery SA, Dunner DL, Dunbar GC (1995) Reduction of suicidal thoughts with paroxetine in comparison with reference antidepressants and placebo. Eur Neuropsychopharmacol 5:5-13
Montgomery SA, Kasper S (1995) Comparison of compliance between serotonin reuptake inhibitors and tricyclic antidepressants: a meta-analysis. Int Clin Psychopharmacol 9 [Suppl 4]:33-40
Muijen M, Roy D, Silverstone T, Mehmet A, Christie M (1988) A comparative clinical trial of fluoxetine, mianserin and placebo with depressed outpatients. Acta Psychiatr Scand 78:384-390
Pande AC, Sayler ME (1993) Adverse events and treatment discontinuations in fluoxetine clinical trials. Int Clin Psychopharmacol 8:267-270
Prien RF, Kupfer DJ (1986) Continuation drug therapy for major depressive episodes: how long should it be maintained? Am J Psychiatry 143:18-23
Song F, Freemantle NS, Sheldon TA, House A, Watson P, Long A (1993) Selective serotonin reuptake inhibitors: meta-analysis of efficacy and acceptability. BMJ 306:683-687
Wakelin JS (1988) The role of serotonin in depression and suicide: do serotonin reuptake inhibitors provide a key? Ad Biol Psychiatry 17:70-83
Wells KB, Stewart A, Hays RD, Burnam MA, Rogers W, Daniels M, Berry S, Greenfield S, Ware CJ (1989) The functioning and well being of depressed patients: results from the medical outcomes study. JAMA 262:914-919
WHO Mental Health Collaborating Centres (1995) Pharmacotherapy of depressive disorders. A consensus statement. J Affect Disord 17:197-198

Negative Symptoms of Schizophrenia: Methodological Issues, Biochemical Findings and Efficacy of Neuroleptic Treatment

H.-J. MÖLLER and M.L. RAO

Introduction

Negative symptoms (minus symptoms) are defined increasingly as a focus of interest both for etiopathogenetic research and psychopharmacological research. However, the findings in both areas are often contradictory, which might be explained by basic methodological problems in the clinical definition and description of the syndrome. Therefore in the first part of this article some of these methodological issues will be shortly reviewed. In the second part a review of biochemical findings will be given. The last part is devoted to the evaluation of the neuroleptic treatment.

Methodological Problems in the Definition and Assessment of Negative Symptoms

A central problem of this scientific approach is that the term "negative symptoms" or "minus symptoms" are not well defined. Different authors use different concepts and definitions for the type and number of symptoms implicated (Helmchen 1988; Rösler and Hengesch 1990). According to Sommers' review, the main negative symptoms concern affect, arousal, cognition, and social functioning (Sommers 1985) and are reflected, for example, by blunted affect, apathy, attentional deficit, poverty of thought or speech, and social withdrawal. Some of these symptoms are elements of the deficit syndrome already described by Bleuler (1911) as "core symptoms" of schizophrenia, or by Huber (1957) as "basic symptoms" of schizophrenia. While some authors support a broad concept of negative symptoms (Gibbons et al. 1985 ; Meltzer and Zureick 1989), others prefer a narrow concept (Strauss et al. 1974; Wing 1978); for instance, Crow (1985) only included flat affect and poverty of speech. The discrepancies particularly concern symptoms such as incoherence, loosening of associations, and thought blocking, which may be interpreted either as negative or as positive symptoms.

The concept of negative symptoms has been refined through factor-analytic studies to better determine whether they are unitary in nature, and the relationship between negative and positive symptoms, i.e., whether they are independent (Lewine et al. 1983) or part of a single dimension, as suggested by Andreasen (1982). When a broad concept of negative symptoms and as a consequence a large number of symptoms have been evaluated, nearly all factor-analytic studies have identified two or three dimensions of negative symptoms (Gibbons et al. 1985; Liddle 1987; Meltzer and Zureick 1989; Gaebel 1993). For example, Meltzer and Zureick (1989) described three factors: cognitive impairment/inappropriate affect, anhedonia/anergia, retardation/flat affect.

The development of special scales like the Scale for the Assessment of Negative Symptoms (SANS; Andreasen 1982) or the Positive and Negative Syndrome Scale (PANSS; Kay et al. 1987) was an important methodological step forward in the measurement of negative symptoms. However, it should be carefully taken into account that there are important differences between these scales, not so much with respect to the general psychopathological areas being covered, but more regarding the selection of items (Zinner et al. 1990; Möller 1991). Such discrepancies become of still more importance if the apathy/anergia/retardation subscales of rating scales commonly used to assess psychotic patients, e. g., the Brief Psychiatric Rating Scale (BPRS), the Inpatient Multidimensional Psychiatric Scale (IMPS), and the rating scale of the Association for Methodology and Documentation in Psychiatry (AMDP), are used to determine negative symptoms.

The lack of homogeneity in the definition and measurement of negative symptoms has potentially important clinical implications. Perhaps some of the inconsistencies in research results can be explained by this fact. Different types of negative symptoms may appear at different stages of schizophrenia or may respond differentially to pharmacological or psychosocial treatments (Meltzer and Zureick 1989; Gaebel 1993).

The differentiation between depression and negative symptoms is difficult on the basis of rating scales (Maier et al. 1990), and therapeutic effects on depressive symptoms might be misinterpreted as successful treatment of negative symptoms and vice versa (Möller 1987). Gaebel (1989) reported a correlation of $r = 0.34 - 0.57$ at different measurement points for the BPRS scores depression and anergia. In our own follow-up study on schizophrenic patients the correlation between the IMPS factor depression and retardation/apathy amounted to $r = 0.35$ (Möller and von Zerssen 1986).

Another problem in the interpretation of rating scale data from studies in this field is that the negative symptoms score correlates positively with the drug-induced Parkinson syndrome (Hoffman et al. 1987; Prosser et al. 1987). Furthermore, there is a correlation between negative symptoms and hyperkinetic neurological symptoms such as akathisia and dyskinesia (Barnes and Braude 1985; Waddington et al. 1985). One could, therefore, conclude that drugs without extrapyramidal side effects in general may appear to be more advantageous in treating negative symptoms (Woggon 1990).

Two recent methodological studies underline these complex interrelationships. A multivariate regression analysis demonstrated that the highest proportion of variance of the negative symptoms score was explained by the variables: depressive symptoms, social adaptation and extrapyramidal symptoms (Bandelow et al. 1990). Gaebel (1990) analyzed in a factor-analytic approach the interactions between depressive symptoms, extrapyramidal symptoms and negative symptoms. Of special importance is that the dimensional structure of a rating system covering all these aspects is not stable during the course of illness.

The differentiation between primary and secondary negative symptoms, as proposed by Carpenter et al. (1985), seems of great relevance. While primary negative symptoms are the consequence of a morbogenic deficit state, e. g., in the sense of type

Table 1. Occurrence of negative symptoms (Angst et al. 1989)

1. In the course of schizophrenia
Prepsychotic period (Conrad 1958; Huber 1957)
Productive psychotic period
Mixture of positive and negative symptoms
Negative symptoms may be hidden
Postpsychotic period
Residuum or defect with or without positive symptoms
Postpsychotic depression, endogenous or reactive (Mayer-Gross 1920)
Postremissive exhaustion (Heinrich 1967)
2. Of other origin
Depression and schizoaffective psychoses
Drug-induced depression
Neuroses and personality disorders
Mild organic brain syndromes
Drug-induced Parkinson syndromes
Institutionalization

II schizophrenia of Crow (1980), secondary negative symptoms are the consequence of: (1) positive symptoms (e.g., social withdrawal because of paranoid ideas); (2) extrapyramidal side effects (e.g., motor retardation as an indicator of akinesia); (3) depressive symptoms (e.g., postpsychotic or pharmacogenic depression); (4) social understimulation (e.g., hospitalism).

According to this theory, the treatment of negative symptoms has to be differentiated concerning the different causes. In a similar direction, Angst et al. (1989) underlined the diagnostic unspecificity of negative symptoms, and listed different kinds of negative symptoms in the course of schizophrenia (Table 1).

In chronic cases, negative symptoms tend to have more stability (Kay and Opler 1987). This led Angst et al. (1989) to assume that drug effects may be more conclusive in the early stage of the disorder. However, with respect to research on drug effects, it has to be considered that, especially in the early stage of schizophrenia, the investigation into neuroleptic treatment of negative symptoms is complicated much more by the instability of the syndrome and by the heterogeneity of causes than in later chronic stages of schizophrenia. Also it has to be considered that it is not the negative symptoms of the acute stage of schizophrenia, in which negative symptoms mostly accompany positive symptoms and have a high chance of disappearing with them, but the negative symptoms of the chronic deficit state which are the greater therapeutic problem.

Crow (1980) postulated the stability of a specific subtype of schizophrenia with positive symptoms (type I) and a subtype with negative symptoms (type II), explaining this by different biological causes. Most other authors stressed the point that negative and positive symptoms can be combined cross-sectionally or longitudinally (Deister et al. 1990) and cannot be taken as indicators for a specific biological or phenomenological subtype.

If one is aware of these principal difficulties in the definition, assessment and ethiopathogenetic typology of negative symptoms, it is not surprising that the biological and psychopharmacological studies are often very controversial in their results. Most of the studies apparently did not take into account all these different problems of the clinical description and differentiation of the phenomenon. Beside differences in the definition (broader vs closer concept) and the assessment procedures (anergy score of the BPRS vs more sophisticated scales like SANS and PANSS), especially the coexistence of negative symptoms with positive symptoms and the lack of differentiation into primary and secondary negative symptoms lead to a lot of difficulties in the interpretation of the data. Therefore it is often difficult to come to clear conclusions concerning the specificity of certain biological findings or of certain treatment procedures.

Biochemical Findings

Several lines of evidence suggest that positive and negative symptoms of schizophrenia differ with respect to morphological, psychobiological and biochemical findings (Andreasen et al. 1982, 1988; Crow 1980; Rao and Möller 1994).

Dopamine

Indirect pharmacologic evidence and results on dopamine metabolite measurements in body fluids suggested that the dopamine turnover, expressed for example as plasma homovanillic acid (HVA), was higher in acutely psychotic patients than in less sick patients (Davidson and Davis 1988; Davis et al. 1985; Maas et al. 1988). However, in schizophrenic patients with negative symptoms, plasma HVA was reduced and the negative symptom score correlated inversely with plasma dopamine metabolite

Table 2. Involvement of reduced dopamine turnover in negative symptoms of schizophrenia (Rao and Möller 1994)

Findings	References
A hypokinetic syndrome occurs in both negative schizophrenia and in Parkinson's disease	(Prosser et al. 1987; Hoffman et al. 1987)
The negative symptom score correlates inversely with plasma HVA concentrations	(Steinberg et al. 1993; Kaminski et al. 1990; Davila et al. 1988)
Lowered HVA excretion is seen predominantly in patients with negative schizophrenia	(Mathieu et al. 1985)
Reduced CSF HVA levels correlate with increased ventricle brain ratios	(Lindström 1985; Nybäck et al. 1983; Losonczy et al. 1986)
Patients with negative symptoms and low plasma HVA concentrations do not show a decrease in HVA on neuroleptic treatment	(Kaminski et al. 1990; Duncan et al. 1993)
Stimulation of dopamine turnover by dopamine agonists improves negative symptoms such as social withdrawal, blunting of affect and motor retardation	(Angrist et al. 1980, 1983)
In patients with negative symptoms there is reduced growth hormone response to the dopamine agonist, apomorphine, compared to patients with positive symptoms	(Zemlan et al. 1986; Meltzer et al. 1984; Ackenheil et al. 1990)

concentrations (HVA) suggesting reduced dopaminergic activity (Table 2) (Steinberg et al. 1993; Kaminski et al. 1990; Davila et al. 1988). Plasma HVA levels rise initially and decline during neuroleptic treatment in responsive schizophrenic patients, but not in treatment refractory schizophrenic patients (Kaminski et al. 1990; Davila et al. 1988; Duncan et al. 1993; Pickar et al. 1986). Therefore, in negative schizophrenia the spontaneously decreased dopaminergic activity precludes a further reduction in the decreased plasma HVA levels by neuroleptic treatment (Kaminski et al. 1990; Duncan et al. 1993). Reduced HVA excretion into the urine was also noted in these patients when compared to age- and sex-matched healthy subjects (Mathieu et al. 1985). Interestingly these relations have been observed although plasma HVA originates as the final metabolic product from central and peripheral catecholaminergic neurons (dopaminergic as well as extraneuronal noradrenergic neurons) and from extraneuronal conversion of DOPA (Kopin 1992). Although only 25% of plasma HVA originates from the brain, data from animals (Bacopoulos et al. 1980; Kendler et al. 1982; Chang et al. 1986) and humans (Kendler et al. 1982a; Davidson et al. 1987; Newcomer et al. 1992) suggest that plasma HVA may be particularly sensitive to changes in central dopaminergic activity.

The finding of reduced dopamine turnover (reduced plasma HVA) is supported by another cue for the putative reduction in dopaminergic neurotransmission, namely decreased cerebrospinal fluid (CSF) HVA. The results on studies with debrisoquin, which inhibits the peripheral catecholamine metabolite formation, indicate that, after blocking peripheral conversion of catecholamines, the CSF HVA levels did not drop (Maas et al. 1985, 1988). In patients with negative symptoms, lowered CSF HVA levels correlated with increased ventricle brain ratios when compared to healthy volunteers (van Kammen et al. 1983; Lindström 1985; Nybäck et al. 1983). These findings are relevant to the behavioral alterations in negative schizophrenia since dopamine is involved in the regulation of performance (D_2 receptors) and reward (D_1 receptors) (Miller et al. 1990).

The MRI of schizophrenic patients shows the increases in the left ventricle to be more extensive than in the right ventricle and the third ventricle of patients to be enlarged compared to healthy subjects (Bogerts et al. 1990). The enlargement was initially attributed to the influence of dopamine D_2 receptor-blocking drugs. However, in several studies drug-naive patients also showed an increase in ventricle volume (Andreasen et al. 1982), chronicity and cortical atrophy (Crow 1985; Pandurangi et al. 1988).

In this context it is of interest that in a condition of reduced dopaminergic activity, i.e., loss of nigrostriatal dopaminergic neurons in Parkinson's disease, a hypokinetic syndrome (akinesia) and anhedonia exist, both of which have also been observed in retarded depression and in negative symptoms of schizophrenia (Bermanzohn and Siris 1992). The notion of dopaminergic dysregulation in retarded depression is based on reduced CSF HVA concentrations, as well as on treatment and challenge studies with dopaminergic agents (Bowers et al. 1969; Goodwin et al. 1973; Insel and Siever 1981; Papeschi and McClure 1971; van Praag and Korf 1973); van Praag and Korf (1973) observed a significant decrease in CSF HVA accumulation in depressed patients with severe motor retardation.

Increased dopamine receptors have been found in post-mortem brains of schizophrenic patients that had been interpreted as linked to hypodopaminergia

(Chouinard and Jones 1978; MacKay 1981; Seeman 1987). This finding has not been duplicated by other groups (Kornhuber et al. 1989) and is not entirely consistent with the observation that dopamine metabolite concentrations in post-mortem brains appear not to be different from controls (Bird et al. 1979). Data on PET analysis of central dopamine D_2 receptors in schizophrenic patients show that the dopamine D_2 receptor densities in the caudate nucleus may be higher in neuroleptic-naive schizophrenic patients compared to healthy subjects which points to receptor up-regulation and supports the notion of functionally lowered dopamine availability (Wong et al. 1986). However, in other studies similar or only slightly increased dopamine D_2 receptor densities were reported (Farde et al. 1987, 1990; König et al. 1991). Studies by Martinot et al. (1990, 1991) suggest that state-dependent fluctuations of the stratal D_2 receptor density were predominated by elevation during the onset or exacerbation of psychotic symptoms, they were not elevated during the chronic course of schizophrenia and did not fall with increasing age as seen in normal controls (Martinot et al. 1991). The putatively decreased dopamine turnover in schizophrenic patients with negative symptoms could be stimulated with the dopamine agonist amphetamine; this was accompanied by an improvement in symptoms such as social withdrawal, blunting of affect and motor retardation (Angrist et al. 1980, 1983; Liebermann et al. 1985; van Kammen and Boronow 1988).

Stimulation of dopamine receptors by the dopamine agonist apomorphine is associated with an increase in growth hormone. This growth hormone response correlated positively with thought disorder and was exaggerated in acute schizophrenia in that the largest growth hormone response was seen in patients who were most psychotic (Zemlan et al. 1986). On the other hand, the decrease in the apomorphine-stimulated release of growth hormone depended on the duration of the disease: it was lower in more chronic patients (Meltzer et al. 1984), in patients with poor premorbid functioning (Zemlan et al. 1986; Ackenheil et al. 1990; Malas et al. 1983), and its outcome correlated with increased negative symptoms (Ferrier et al. 1984). Taken together, these data suggest diverging alterations in the dopaminergic systems in schizophrenic subgroups, i.e., a decrease in dopamine tumover during negative and an increase during positive symptomatology.

Norepinephrine

Analogous to dopamine, the increase in norepinephrine turnover correlated with psychotic symptoms (Linnoila et al. 1983). Disturbances in the noradrenergic transmission are accompanied by those of the autonomic system and are seen conjointly with negative symptoms, such as a deficit of attention and a disturbance in information processing (van Kammen and Antelman 1984). Thus, positive symptoms seem to be related to an overactivity in the noradrenergic system and negative symptoms of schizophrenia to a reduction in the norepinephrine turnover (Gelernter and van Kammen 1990). This contention was supported by the observation that norepinephrine was elevated in the limbic system of paranoid schizophrenics (Farley et al. 1980).

As for the norepinephrine levels in the brain, the results are not unanimous since similar (Kleinmann et al. 1979), increased (Crow et al. 1979) and decreased (Nybäck et al. 1983) norepinephrine levels were found in post-mortem schizophrenic brains compared to those of healthy subjects. The incidence of negative symptoms in schizophrenia is difficult to assess since these case histories do not give any data on

Table 3. Involvement of reduced norepinephrine or serotonin turnover in negative symptoms of schizophrenia (Rao and Möller 1994)

Findings	References
Norepinephrine	
Reduced CSF norepinephrine and MHPG levels have been observed in negative schizophrenia	(van Kammen et al. 1991)
Increased MAO activity is associated with negative symptoms and with low catecholamine levels	(Lewine and Meltzer 1984)
Decreased CSF dopamine-β-hydroxylase activity is associated with increased ventricle-to-brain ratios in patients with negative schizophrenia (for details see text)	(van Kammen et al. 1983)
Reduced α_2 adrenoceptor activity on platelets and in brain have been found in schizophrenia	(Rosen et al. 1985)
Serotonin	
Ventricle enlargement and chronicity are accompanied by decreased serotonin turnover	(Gelernter and van Kammen 1990)
The negative symptom score and cortical atrophy correlate inversely with low CSF 5-HIAA concentrations	(Potkin et al. 1983; Losonczy et al. 1986)

the proportion of patients with negative symptoms. However, as regards CSF, van Kammen et al. (1991) observed decreased norepinephrine and MHPG concentrations in schizophrenic patients with negative symptoms (Table 3).

It was speculated that the disturbance in noradrenergic and dopaminergic transmission could be due to perturbation of dopamine β-hydroxylase activity. Stein and Wise (1971) proposed that a functional deficit of dopamine β-hydroxylase activity might increase the overflow of dopamine from noradrenergic nerve endings. Dopamine, when hydroxylated to the neurotoxin 6-hydroxydopamine, might regain entry into neurons, destroy noradrenergic neurons and thus produce the burnt-out syndrome of schizophrenia. Dopamine β-hydroxylase is liberated when norepinephrine is released into the synaptic cleft and circulates in CSF and serum. Van Kammen et al. (1983) related CSF HVA and CSF dopamine β-hydroxylase to normal and abnormal CT scans and found decreased CSF concentrations of HVA and decreased dopamine β-hydroxylase activity to be associated with increased ventricle-to-brain ratios. The reduction in dopamine β-hydroxylase might also be related to the reduced norepinephrine turnover in this condition. The results are far from clear-cut since the dopamine β-hydroxylase activity did not correlate with the clinical subtype of schizophrenia (Gelernter and van Kammen 1990).

On the other hand, it has been observed in the animal model that norepinephrine interacts with dopamine D_1 (van der Heyden et al. 1986) and dopamine D_2 receptors (Swerdlow and Koob 1989). The link between the two receptor systems is thought to be via α_2 receptors (Reubenstein et al. 1989; Delini and Hunn 1990; Dickinson et al. 1988). In this respect it is of interest that various antidepressant treatment modalities down-regulate the α_2 adrenoreceptor activity in platelets and in the brain in a similar fashion and this down-regulation is comparable to the onset of clinical efficacy in depressed patients (Smith et al. 1981; Cohen et al. 1982; Pilc and Vetulani 1982; Piletz et al. 1986, 1991). Piletz et al. (1986) pointed out that the investigations of platelet adrenoreceptors in humans are not entirely consistent, but some of these inconsistencies have been traced to different methodology and different ligands. Although there is little such information on schizophrenic patients with negative symptoms, a decrease in the number of α_2 receptor-binding sites on thrombocytes has been noted (Rosen et al. 1985).

Serotonin

Serotonin's involvement in schizophrenia has been indirectly inferred from the observation that the hallucinogen LSD interacts with serotonin receptors (Gaddum 1954). This led to the "transmethylation" theory of schizophrenia, which has proved controversial, since no alterations in methylated indoleamines were found in body fluids (Carpenter et al. 1975; Axelsson and Nordgren 1974) and since the perceptual disturbances observed after LSD were rarely seen in schizophrenia (Snyder 1972). However, serotonergic networks may be involved in the negative symptomatology, since ventricle enlargement and chronicity were accompanied in schizophrenic patients by decreased serotonin turnover (Gelernter and van Kammen 1990).

Little is known on the interaction of serotonin and dopamine in the brain. It is conceivable that because of the increased dopamine turnover in cases of positive symptoms and of decreased dopamine turnover in those of negative symptoms of schizophrenia, serotonergic neuronal activity may be differentially expressed and thus may be state-dependent. Post-mortem brain studies on schizophrenic patients, which were not broken down into groups of previous positive and negative symptom episodes, yielded contradictory results with respect to the concentration of serotonin, its precursors, metabolites and central receptors (Gelernter and van Kammen 1990). The majority of studies showed similar concentrations of the CSF serotonin metabolite 5-hydroxyindoleacetic acid (5-HIAA) between schizophrenic patients and controls (Persson and Roos 1969; Rimon et al. 1971; Post et al. 1975; Nybäck et al. 1983; Potkin et al. 1983). However, in subgroups of schizophrenics the concentrations of the CSF 5-HIAA correlated negatively with cortical atrophy (Table 3) (Gelernter and van Kammen 1990; Losonczy et al. 1986). Thus a concurrence between serotonergic deficiency in the prefrontal cortex and negative symptoms of schizophrenia has been postulated (Bleich et al. 1988).

The Efficacy of Neuroleptics in Negative Symptoms

There is a strong debate in the literature, whether neuroleptics are able to reduce negative symptoms and whether this is a direct or an indirect (e.g. via reduction of positive symptoms) effect (Möller 1993).

Classical Neuroleptics

Crow (1980) based his hypothesis on the nonresponsiveness of negative symptoms mainly on his work with Johnstone et al. (1978) and the studies of Angrist et al. (1980). Johnstone et al. (1978) carried out a 4-week double-blind trial using placebo, α-flupenthixol and β-flupenthixol in 45 acute schizophrenics. There were no differences with respect to negative symptoms of the α-isomer (active neuroleptic) compared with the placebo and β-isomer (inactive). Flattening of affect and poverty of speech were not improved with neuroleptics, nor were the items for depression, anxiety and retardation. The study was criticized by Ashcroft et al. (1981) and Meltzer (1985) under different aspects: too low baseline scores of negative symptoms, too small sample size, too short duration of the trial and too low dosage of α-flupenthixol. Angrist et al. (1980) treated 21 schizophrenics (10 acute or subacute and 11 chronic or subchronic) with 'large doses' of neuroleptics and amphetamines in an attempt to confirm Crow's model. Positive symptoms (thought disturbances, activation and hostile suspiciousness, BPRS factors) were diminished by neuroleptics and increased by amphetamines. The withdrawal/retardation factor was not affected by neuroleptics.

In his review, Goldberg (1985) cited five large placebo-controlled studies to demonstrate that contrary to the contention of Johnstone et al. (1976) and Crow (1980), negative and/or deficit symptoms in schizophrenia do indeed respond to neuroleptic treatment. He described, for example, the NIMH collaborative group studies on phenothiazines, where, highly significant drug-placebo differences were shown in a variety of "positive, negative and deficit schizophrenic symptoms." Included in the latter two categories are: indifference to environment or apathy, hebephrenic symptoms or inappropriate affect, slowed speech and movements, poor social participation, and poor self-care and confusion. According to his review, the greater drug effects were shown in 'negative' symptoms like hebephrenic symptoms, poor social participatiom confusion, and poor self-care rather than positive symptoms. He differentiated this observation, however, by stating that without subtracting the placebo effect, the negative or deficit symptoms do not change as much as the positive symptoms (Table 4). Goldberg (1985) also quoted the review by Cole et al. (1966) as a proof of his hypothesis. In this summary of other controlled studies on phenothiazines too, similar results were found. Two of the studies demonstrated a reduction in blunted affect and indifference. Four of the studies showed an effect on withdrawal/retardation, and four of the studies showed a drug effect on autistic behavior and mannerisms. Several problems of interpreting such data that have already been discussed have to be taken into account. For example, it has to be stated that all these studies were performed in acute schizophrenic patients, and the definition of negative symptoms seems very broad when hebephrenic symptoms, confusion, and mannerisms are included in this concept.

Table 4. Greater reduction of negative and/or deficit symptoms under drug than placebo (Goldberg 1985)

	Placebo pre: post change standard scores	Drug pre: post change standard scores	P
Indifference to environment (n = 214)	0.353	1.234	<0.01
Slowed speech and movements (n = 245)	0.114	0.849	<0.01
Social participation vs. withdrawal (n = 302)	0.788	1.776	<0.01
Hebephrenic symptoms (n = 150)	0.247	1.437	<0.01
Confusion (n = 276)	0.620	1.600	<0.01
Poor self-care (n = 224)	0.349	1.283	<0.01

Meltzer et al. (1986) also stated that negative symptoms respond to conventional neuroleptics and tried to support this opinion with a study (Meltzer 1985). Meltzer (1985) studied schizophrenic inpatients treated for an average of 10 weeks (5–15 weeks) with neuroleptics (and other agents) to demonstrate the change in negative symptoms in a clinical setting. An 11-item negative symptom scale was used. Significant improvement between admission and discharge in both positive and negative symptoms (more significant in women) was found. In 21 of 55 patients (38%) with extensive negative scores, the improvement was substantial. Using an analysis of covariance, they tried to demonstrate that improvement in negative symptoms was more than an indirect effect of the improvement of positive symptoms. Unfortunately, this naturalistic study cannot control the effects of placebo conditions or other treatment factors.

In a similar investigation on a large sample of schizophrenic inpatients treated under routine care conditions, mostly with haloperidol as treatment of first choice, we found that not only productive symptoms, but also symptoms of the depressive-apathic spectrum were reduced between admission and discharge (Möller and von Zerssen, 1981, 1982, 1986). Especially the IMPS factor 'retardation and apathy' can be interpreted as an indicator of negative symptoms.

Gaebel (1993) reported differential effects on the spectrum of negative symptoms, comparing perazine and haloperidol. While the productive symptoms and most SANS dimensions demonstrated no difference between the two neuroleptics, a therapeutic superiority of perazine was observed with respect to flat affect. Breier et al. (1987) used a double-blind placebo-controlled design to evaluate the effect of neuroleptics on negative symptoms. They scored 19 chronic schizophrenics with the Scale of Emotional Blunting (SEB; Abrams and Taylor, 1978) and the BPRS. The neuroleptic withdrawal produced a significant increase in negative symptom scores on both scales. The 4 weeks of neuroleptic treatment led to a decrease in score on both scales. The relationship between changes of positive and negative symptoms was not analyzed.

Diphenylbutylpiperidines and Benzamides

Different groups proposed that diphenylbutylpiperidines are more effective than other neuroleptics in the treatment of schizophrenic negative symptoms (Pinder et al. 1976; Gould et al. 1983). This was explained, among other, by the lack of a noradrenergic receptor blockade under the hypothesis that the blockade of the noradrenergic receptors induces sedation and an unfavorable influence of the central noradrenergic reward system which could cause negative symptoms. It was also suggested that the specific action is related to the blockage of voltage-operated calcium channels, but there is little evidence to support this hypothesis from studies on calcium antagonists like verapamil which had not been found to have antischizophrenic properties (Grebb et al. 1982; Pickar et al. 1987).

Pinder et al. (1976) reviewed 22 double-blind studies – most of them not specifically designed to investigate the therapeutic effect on negative symptoms – comparing pimozide with other neuroleptics. In only 10 studies individual BPRS items were clearly specified and in most of these, both pimozide and the standard neuroleptics were effective in decreasing emotional withdrawal, blunted affect and motor retardation. Only in two studies (Andersen et al. 1974; Kolivakis et al. 1974) pimozide did better than the comparator in emotional withdrawal or psychomotor retardation items. Nevertheless, the authors came to the general conclusion that pimozide may be superior to other neuroleptics in improving psychomotor retardation and emotional withdrawal. The review of De Leon and Simpson (1991) summarized the results on nine more recently published double-blind studies comparing pimozide with other neuroleptics. Six studies with a prolonged treatment period in chronic schizophrenics are perhaps more important for addressing the stability of negative symptoms, but these studies in general gave no evidence for an advantage of pimozide. In only one of these studies (Abuzzahab and Zimmermann 1980) pimozide was shown to be superior to fluphenazine in the withdrawal/retardation factor. In two of these three studies which used pimozide in higher dosages in acute schizophrenia, there was a tendency for pimozide to be more effective for psychomotor retardation or anergia (Chouinard and Annable 1982; Haas and Beckmann 1982). However, in both studies pimozide patients received more anticholinergic medication for treatment of extrapyramidal side effects than those treated with the comparators.

These control-group studies raise the questions whether pimozide really has an effect on negative symptoms or is only favorable insofar as it does not induce as much sedation, apathy or akinesia as chlorpromazine or fluphenazine. Also the question whether the dosages in the experimental and control groups were really equivalent should be discussed.

In a more recently published placebo-controlled study on pimozide (van Kammen et al. 1987), the neuroleptic treatment did not exert a differential effect on the positive and negative symptoms of schizophrenia. Both groups of symptoms responded. Changes in the positive and negative symptoms of schizophrenia were directly related: "Thus, patients whose hallucinations, delusions and disorganized speech improved during neuroleptic treatment also became less withdrawn, emotionally flat and motorically slowed" (van Kammen et al. 1987). This statement could support the hypothesis that secondary negative symptoms in the sense of Carpenter were responsive.

For the other diphenylbutylpiperidines – penfluridol and fluspirilene – the situation is quite similar to that with pimozide, as the review by De Leon and Simpson (1991) demonstrated. In these studies there was no difference between penfluridol or fluspirilene and the comparators with respect to negative symptoms. In one double-blind study penfluridol was reported to be more effective in reducing the anergia factor (Gallant et al. 1974). In one study comparing fluspirilene with fluphenazine decanoate (Malm et al. 1974) an advantage with respect to negative symptoms was found but perhaps the inferior result of fluphenazine has to be explained under the aspect of more side effects in the fluphenazine group.

The benzamides have also been described as advantageous with respect to negative symptoms. Hitherto, most data have been collected for sulpiride (De Leon and Simpson 1991) (Table 5). The evidence for a specific antiautistic activity of sulpiride comes fundamentally from open trials (Peselow and Stanley 1982). Although earlier double-blind trials seem to support this hypothesis, the results have to be questioned because of severe methodological problems (Edwards et al. 1980). The more recent and better designed double-blind trials were reviewed by De Leon and Simpson (1991) (see Table 5). Most of them did not show any specific effect for sulpiride on negative symptoms. Only one study out of four suggested a specific antiautistic

Table 5. Sulpiride versus other neuroleptic double-blind studies (De Leon and Simpson 1991)

Reference	Patient type	Diagnosis	Dosage (mg/day)	Other NL	Duration (months)	Differential effect of sulpiride				Comments
						On NS	On PS	Parkinsonian S	On SocNurSC	
Edwards et al. (1980)	Chronic (38)	FRS or/and FTD	600–1800	Trifluoperazine 15–45	1.5	=	=	=	Not Used	
Rao et al. (1981)	Chronic (30)	Non-sp. European	1200	Haloperidol 10 (5–40)	3	=	=	<	= WWBS	
Gerlach et al. (1985)	Chronic (20)	Feighner	2000 (800–3200)	Haloperidol 12 (6–24)	3	=	Non-sp.	< In 4 1st weeks	Not used	
Härnryd et al. (1984)	Acute (50)	RDC	800	Chlorpromazine 400	2	=	=	<NS	<RS NOSIE	Due to worsening of CPZ patients

FRS, first rank symptoms of Schneider; FTD, formal thought disturbance; Non-sp, non-specified; NOSIE, Nurses Observation Scale for Inpatient Evaluations; NS, nonsignificant; On NS, effect on negative symptoms; On PS, effect on positive symptoms; On SocNurSC, social or nursing scales. (>: sulpiride had greater effect; <: sulpiride had lower effect; Parkinsonian S, parkinsonian symptoms (>: sulpiride induced more; <: sulpiride induced less); RS, retardation subscale; WWBS, Wing Ward Behavior Scale

activity on one scale and this was probably due to fewer extrapyramidal symptoms. Recently, remoxipride, another benzamide, was introduced on the market. It can be characterized from the pharmacological viewpoint as a selective D_2 antagonist with a preferential mesolimbic mode of action and from the clinical viewpoint as an atypical neuroleptic (a neuroleptic with a comparatively low frequency of extrapyramidal side effects). In a double-blind study on acute schizophrenics, remoxipride was more effective than haloperidol in reducing negative symptoms (Laux et al. 1990).

Clozapine and D_2-S_2 Antagonists

The strongest body of evidence which supports the ability of atypical antipsychotic drugs to improve negative symptoms seems available from studies of clozapine (Müller-Spahn 1990; Meltzer 1991). Clozapine is often classified as an atypical neuroleptic to underline that it lacks the risk of extrapyramidal side effects.

Claghorn et al. (1987) reported that clozapine was significantly more effective than chlorpromazine in reducing BPRS anergia/withdrawal ratings in 150 schizophrenic patients with tardive dyskinesia or moderate to severe extrapyramidal symptoms who were randomly assigned to either treatment. Patients who had been chronically hospitalized were excluded. Both at 8 weeks and with an endpoint analysis, the improvement in this factor with clozapine, compared with chlorpromazine treatment, was greater than that for any other BPRS factor. This was true despite the fact that the two drugs were equivalent in improving motor retardation. Nurses' ratings supported the superiority of clozapine in improving social function.

The study of Kane et al. (1988) examined the efficacy of clozapine in treatment-resistant schizophrenic patients. A total of 305 schizophrenic patients with a history of failure to respond to at least three neuroleptics of two different classes were included. In the first phase, these patients were treated with high doses of haloperidol for 6 weeks. Less than 2% responded. The nonresponders plus a small group of haloperidol-intolerant patients were then randomly assigned to clozapine or chlorpromazine plus an anticholinergic drug for 6 weeks. Clozapine was superior to chlorpromazine in decreasing BPRS positive symptoms from weeks 1 to 6: BPRS anergia/withdrawal showed greater improvement in the clozapine than the chlorpromazine group between weeks 2 and 6. Significantly greater improvement in social function in the clozapine group was noted in the nurses' rating.

Meltzer et al. (1989) reported preliminary results of an open, prospective study of the effect of clozapine in 51 treatment-resistant schizophrenic patients under long-term conditions. These patients were described as similar in severity to those studied by Kane et al. (1988). The duration of treatment with clozapine was 1.5–35.2 months (mean 10.3 months). Significant decreases were noted in the BPRS withdrawal/retardation scale, with increasing improvement over time. An analysis of covariance demonstrated that the improvement in BPRS withdrawal/retardation ratings was independent of improvement in positive symptoms.

Meanwhile data are available on 85 patients whose treatment with clozapine was begun 12 months prior to the point of data analysis. The results are similar to the subgroup investigated earlier (Meltzer 1991).

With respect to its pharmacological profile clozapine can be characterized as a D_2-S_2 antagonist. A double-blind study comparing the D_2-S_2 antagonist zotepine with perazine did not prove zotepine to be superior with respect to negative symptoms (Müller-Spahn 1991). In both groups the amelioration of the SANS scores was similar.

Another more potent D_2-S_2 receptor-antagonist, risperidone, recently developed, could demonstrate in schizophrenic patients advantages in negative symptoms, especially in comparison with haloperidol. Evidence for this was especially given in the so called North American Study, comparing different dosages of risperidone with haloperidol and placebo (Marder and Meibach 1994). It was shown, by a path-analytical approach, that the superiority of risperidone concerning negative symptoms is not only due to a superiority in reducing positive symptoms or due to a more favorable extrapyramidal side effects profile. In the path-analytical calculation it could be proven that after out-partialisation of these both effects, there remains still a direct effect (Möller et al. 1995; Fig. 1). This statistical approach seems to be advisable for getting more insight in the problem whether a neuroleptic acts directly or indirectly on negative symptoms. However there is also the need for better clinical trials in this field (Möller et al. 1994; Table 6).

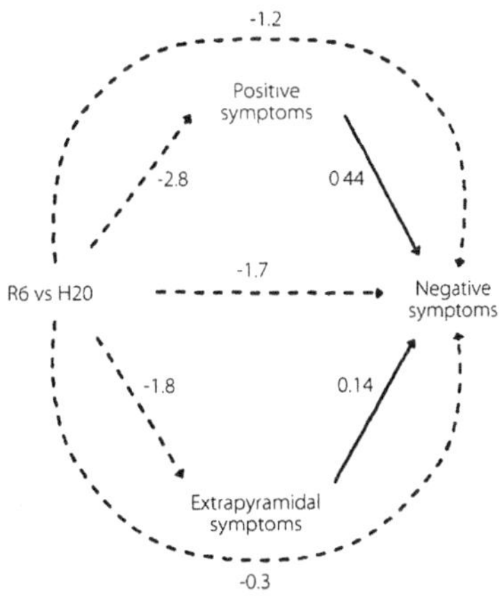

Fig. 1. Estimated path coefficients for the comparison of 6 mg risperidone (R6) ($n = 85$) and 20 mg haloperidol (H20) ($n = 85$). *Continuous lines* denote equally directed relationships, *dashed lines* inverse relationships; the *semicircles* represent the indirect effects of the treatment; all parameters are significant ($p < 0.05$)

Table 6. Suggetions of the working group on negative symptoms in schizophrenia (Möller et al. 1994)

Aim: Evaluation of treatment effects on negative symptoms in schizophrenia

1. Patient selection:
   (a) Positive symptoms not dominating the actual clinical picture, e.g., PANSS negative type
   (b) Duration of negative symptoms > 6 months
   (c) Stable condition of the schizophrenic illness > 6 months
   (d) Flat affect and poverty of speech as core symptoms of negative symptoms
   (e) No/low depression score
2. Design: double-blind comparison to placebo or active drug
3. Efficacy parameters: BPRS or SANS or PANSS
4. Other scales: depression scales, EPS scales
5. Statistical analyses:
   (a) End point comparison
   (b) Interaction with productive symptoms, depression, EPS

Summary

The most prominent biochemical finding in schizophrenic patients with negative symptoms appears to be the reduction of central dopaminergic, serotonergic and noradrenergic activities. This decrease in amine activity tends to be associated with structural brain abnormalities, i.e. cortical atrophy or enlarged ventricles. However these findings are somewhat controversial and because of several methodological problems it seems difficult to come to a clear conclusion.

Negative symptoms accompanying productive symptoms do improve with the neuroleptic treatment of the productive symptoms. However it is questionable whether neuroleptics in general are effective in primary negative symptoms. Most data from controlled studies are not totally conclusive because of several methodological pitfalls. There are very few studies which try to differentiate between the direct and the indirect (via reduction of positive symptoms or via a better extrapyramidal tolerability) effect of neuroleptics on negative symptoms. The application of sophisticated statistical procedures can help to get insight into this problem.

References

Abbuzzahab Zimmermann RL (1980) Factors determining patient tenure on a 3-year double-blind investigation of pimozide versus fluphenazine HCI. Adv Biochem Psychopharmacol 24: 547–550

Abrams Taylor MA (1978) A rating scale for emotional blunting. Am J Psychiatry 135:226–229

Ackenheil M, Bondy B, Müller-Spahn F (1990) Biochemische und neuroendokrinologische Befunde bei Patienten mit schizophrener Minus-symptomatik. In: Möller HJ, Pelzer E (eds) Neuere Ansätze zur Diagnostik und Therapie schizophrener Minussymptomatik. Springer, Berlin Hedelberg New York pp 127–134

Andersen K, D'Elia G, Hallberg B, Perris C, Rapp W, Roman G (1974) A controlled trial of pimozide and trifluoperazine and chronic schizophrenic syndromes. Acta Psychiatr Scand 50 Suppl 240:43–64

Andreasen NC (1982) Negative symptoms in schizophrenia: definition and reliability. Arch Gen Psychiatry 39:784–788

Andreasen NC, Smith MR, Jacoby CG, Dennert JW, Olsen SA (1982) Ventricular enlargement in schizophrenia: definition and prevalence. Am J Psychiatry 139:292–296

Andreasen NC, Carson R, Diksic M, Evans A, Farde L, Gjedde A, Hakim A, Samarthji L, Nair N, Sedvall G, Tune L, Wong D (1988) Workshop on schizophrenia, PET, and dopamine D_2 receptors in the human neostriatum. Schizophr Bull 14:471–484

Angrist B, Rotrosen J, Gershon S (1980) Differential effects of amphetamine and neuroleptics on negative versus positive symptoms in schizophrenia. Psychopharmacolog (Berl) 72:17–19

Angrist B, Peselow E, Rubinstein M, Corwin J, Rotrosen J (1983) Partial improvement in negative schizophrenic symptoms after amphetamine. Psychopharmacology (Berl) 78:128–130

Angst J, Stassen HH, Woggon B (1989) Effect of neuroleptics on positive and negative symptoms and the deficit state. Psychopharmacology (Berl) 99:41–46

Ashcroft GW, Blackwood GW, Besson JAO, Palomo T, Waring HL (1981) Positive and negative schizophrenic symptoms and the role of dopamine. Br J Psychiatry 138:268–269

Axelsson S, Nordgren L (1974) Indoleamines in blood plasma of schizophrenics: a critical study with sensitive and selective methods. Life Sci 14:1261–1270

Bacopoulos NG, Redmond DE, Baulu J, Roth RH (1980) Chronic haloperidol or fluphenazine: effects on dopamine metabolism in brain, cerebrospinal fluid and plasma of *Ceropithecus aethiops* (vervet monkey). J Pharmacol Exp Ther 212:1–5

Bandelow B, Müller P, Gaebel W, Köpcke W, Linden M, Müller-Spahn F, Pietzcker A, Reischies FM, Tegeler J (1990) Depressive syndromes in schizophrenic patients after discharge from hospital. Eur Arch Psychiatry Clin Neurosci 240:113-120
Barnes TR, Braude WM (1985) Akathisia variants and tardive dyskinesia. Arch Gen Psychiatry 42:874-878
Bermanzohn PC, Siris SG (1992) Akinesia: syndrome common to parkinsonism, retarded depression, and negative symptoms of schizophrenia. Compr Psychiatry 33:221-232
Bird ED, Crow TJ, Iversen LL, Longden A, MacKay AVP, Riley GJ, Spokes EG (1979) Dopamine and homovanillic acid concentration in post-mortem brain in schizophrenia. J Physiol (Lond) 293:36-37
Bleich A, Brown SL, Kahn R, van Praag HM (1988) The role of serotonin in schizophrenia. Schizophr Bull 14:297-315
Bleuler E (1911) Dementia praecox oder Gruppe der Schizophrenien. In: Aschaffenburg G (ed) Handbuch der Psychiatrie. Deuticke, Leipzig, pp 1-420
Bogerts B, Falkai P, Degreef G, Ashtari M, Lieberman J (1990) Postmortale und kernspintomographische Untersuchungen an schizophrenen Patienten - Korrelation mit schizophrener Plus- und Minussymptomatik. In: Möller HJ, Pelzer E (eds) Neuere Ansätze zur Diagnostik und Therapie schizophrener Minussymptomatik. Springer, Berlin Heidelberg New York, pp 103-112
Bowers MB Jr, Heninger GR, Gerbode F (1969) Cerebrospinal fluid 5- hydroxyindolacetic acid and homovanillic acid in psychiatric patients. Int J Neuropharmacol 8:255-262
Breier A, Wolkowitz OM, Doran AR, Roy A, Boronow J, Hommer DW, Pickar D (1987) Neuroleptic responsivity of negative and positive symptoms in schizophrenia. Am J Psychiatry 144:1549-1555
Carpenter WT Jr, Fink EB, Narasimhachari N, Himwich H (1975) A test of the transmethylation hypothesis in acute schizophrenic patients. Am J Psychiatry 132:1261-1270
Carpenter WT, Heinrichs DW, Alphs LD (1985) Treatment of negative symptoms. Schizophr Bull 11:440-452
Chang WH, Yeh EK, Hu WH, Tseng YT, Chung MC, Chang HF (1986) Acute and chronic effects of haloperidol on plasma and brain homovanillic acid in the rat. Biol Psychiatry 21:374-381
Chouinard G, Annable L (1982) Pimozide in the treatment of newly admitted schizophrenic patients. Psychopharmacology (Berl) 76:13-19
Chouinard G, Jones BD (1978) Schizophrenia as a dopamine defficiency disease. Lancet 2:99-100
Claghorn J, Honigfeld G, Abuzzahab PS, Wang R, Steinbook R, Tuason V, Klerman G (1987) The risks and benefits of clozapine versus chlorpromazine. J Clin Psychopharmacol 7:377-384
Cohen RM, Ebstein RP, Daly JW, Murphy DL (1982) Chronic effects of a monoamine oxidase-inhibiting antidepressant: decreases in functional alpha-adrenergic autoreceptors precede the decrease in norepinephrine-stimulated cyclic 3', 5'-monophosphate systems in rat brain. J Neurosci 2:1588-1595
Cole JO, Goldberg SC, Davis JM (1966) Drugs in the treatment of psychosis: Controlled studies. In: Solomon P (ed) Psychiatric drugs. Grune and Stratton, New York, pp 153-180
Conrad K (1958) Die beginnende Schizophrenie. Thieme, Stuttgart
Crow TJ (1980) Molecular pathology of schizophrenia: more than one disease process? Br Med J 280:66-68
Crow TJ (1985) The two syndrome concept: origins and current status. Schizophr Bull 11:471-486
Crow TJ, Baker HF, Cross AJ, Joseph MH, Lofthouse R, Longden A, Owen F, Riley GJ, Glover V, Killpack WS (1979) Monoamine mechanisms in chronic schizophrenia: post mortem neurochemical findings. Br J Psychiatry 134:249-256
Davidson M, Davis KL (1988) A comparison of plasma homovanillic acid concentrations in schizophrenic and normal controls. Arch Gen Psychiatry 45:561-563
Davidson M, Losonczy MF, Mohs RC, Lessre JC, Powchik P, Freed LB, Davis KL (1987) Effects of debrisoquin and haloperidol on plasma homovanillic acid in schizophrenic patients. Neuropsychopharmacology 1:17-23
Davila R, Manero E, Zumarraga AI, Schweitzer JW, Friedhoff AJ (1988) Plasma homovanillic acid as a predictor of response to neuroleptics. Arch Gen Psychiatry 45:564-567
Davis KL, Davidson M, Mohs RC, Kendler KS, Davis BM, Johns CA, Denigris Y, Hovath TB (1985) Plasma homovanillic acid concentration and the severety of schizophrenic illness. Science 227:1601-1602
De Leon J, Simpson GM (1991) Do schizophrenic negative symptoms respond to neuroleptics? Integr Psychiatry 7:39-47
Deister A, Marneros A, Rohde A (1990) Zur Stabilität negativer und positiver Syndromatik. In: Möller HJ, Pelzer E (eds) Neuere Ansätze zur Diagnostik und Therapie schizophrener Minussymptomatik. Springer, Berlin Heidelberg New York, pp 25-34

Delini A, Hunn C (1990) Effects of single and repeated treatment with antidepressants on apomorphine-induced yawning in the rat. The implications of alpha-1-adrenergic mechanisms in the D_2-receptor function. Psychopharmacology (Berl) 101:62-66
Dickinson SL, Gadie B, Tulloch IF (1988) Alpha-1- and alpha-2-adrenoreceptor antagonists differentially influence locomotor and stereotyped behavior induced by *d*-amphetamine and apomorphine in the rat. Psychopharmacology (Berl) 96:521-527
Duncan E, Wolkin A, Angrist B, Sanfilipo M, Wieland S, Cooper TB, Rotrosen J (1993) Plasma homovanillic acid in neuroleptic responsive and nonresponsive schizophrenics. Biol Psychiatry 34:523-528
Edwards JG, Alexander JR, Alexander MS, Gordon A, Zutchi D (1980) Controlled trial of sulpiride in chronic schizophrenic patients. Br J Psychiatry 137:522-529
Farde L, Wiesel FA, Hall H, Halldin C, Stone-Elander S, Sedvall G (1987) No D_2 receptor increase in PET study of schizophrenia. Arch Gen Psychiatry 44:671-672
Farde L, Wiesel FA, Stone-Elander S, Halldin C, Norström AL, Hall H, Sedvall G (1990) D_2-dopamine receptors in neuroleptic-naive schizophrenic patients. Arch Gen Psychiatry 47:213-219
Farley I, Shannak K, Hornykiewicz D (1980) Brain momoamine changes in chronic paranoid schizophrenia and their possible relation to increased dopamine receptor sensitivity. In: Pepeu G, Kuhar M, Enna S (eds) Receptors for neurotransmitters and peptide hormones. Raven, New York, pp 427-433
Ferrier IN, Crow TJ, Roberts GW, Johnstone EC, Owens DGC, Lee Y, Baracese-Hamilton A, McGregor G, O'Shoughnessy D, Polak JM, Bloom SR (1984) Clinical effects of apomorphine in schizophrenia. In: Trimble M, Zarafian E (eds) Psychopharmacology of the lymbic system. Oxford University Press, Oxford (BPA monograph no 5)
Gaddum JH (1954) Drugs antagonistic to 5-hydroxytryptamine. In: Wolstenholme GW (ed) Ciba Foundation symposium on hypertension. Little Brown, Boston, pp 75-77
Gaebel W (1989) Indikatoren und Prädiktoren schizophrener Krankheitsstadien und Verlaufsausgänge. *Habilitationsschrift*, Freie University of Berlin
Gaebel W (1990) Erfassung und Differenzierung schizophrener Minussymptomatik mit objektiven verhaltensanalytischen Methoden. In: Möller HJ, Pelzer F (eds) Neuere Ansätze zur Diagnostik und Therapie schizophrener Minussymptomatik. Springer, Berlin Heidelberg New York, pp 79-90
Gaebel W (1993) Parkinsonoid, Akinese, negative und depressive Symptomatik bei schizophrenen Erkrankungen. In: Möller HJ, Przuntek H (eds) Therapie im Grenzgebiet von Psychiatrie und Neurologie. Springer, Berlin Heidelberg New York
Gallant DM, Mielke DH, Spirtes MA, Swanson WC, Bost R (1974) Penfluoridol: an efficacious long-acting oral antipsychotic compound. Am J Psychiatry 131:699-702
Gelernter J, van Kammen DP (1990) Schizophrenia: instability in norepinephrine, serotonin and γ-aminobutyric acid systems. Int Rev Neurobiol 29:309-347
Gerlach J, Behnke K, Heltberg J, Munk-Andersen E, Nielsen H (1985) Sulpiride and haloperidol in schizophrenia: a double-blind cross-over study of therapeutic effect, side effects and plasma concentrations. Br J Psychiatry 147: 283-288
Gibbons RD, Lewine RRJ, Davis JM, Schooler NR, Cole JO (1985) An empirical test of a Kraepelinian vs a Bleulerian view of negative symptoms. Schizophr Bull 11:390-396
Goldberg SC (1985) Negative and deficit symptoms in schizophrenia do respond to neuroleptics. Schizophr Bull 11:453-456
Goodwin F, Post R, Dunner D, Gordon EK (1973) Cerebrospinal fluid amine metabolites in affective illness. Am J Psychiatry 130:73-79
Gould RJ, Murray KMM, Reynolds JJ, Snyder SH (1983) Antischizophrenic drugs of the diphenylbutylpiperidine type act as calcium channel antagonists. Proc Natl Acad Sci USA 80:5122-5125
Grebb JA, Shelton RC, Taylor EH, Bigelow LB (1982) A negative, double-blind, placebo-controlled, clinical trial of verapamil in chronic schizophrenia. Biol Psychiatry 21: 691-694
Haas S, Beckmann H (1982) Pimozide versus haloperidol in acute schizophrenia. A double blind controlled study. Pharmacopsychiatry 15:70-74
Härnryd C, Bjerkenstedt L, Björk K, Gullberg B, Oxenstierna G, Sedvall G, Wiesel FA, Wik G, Aberg-Wistedt A (1984) Clinical evaluation of sulpiride in schizophrenic patients: a double-blind comparison with chlorpromazine. Acta Psychiatr Scand. Suppl 311: 7-30
Heinrich K (1967) Zur Bedeutung des postremissiven Erschöpfungssyndroms für die Rehabilitation Schizophrener. Nervenarzt 38:487-491
Helmchen H (1988) Methodologische und strategische Erwägungen in der Schizophrenie-Forschung. Fortschr Neurol Psychiatr 56:379-389

Hoffman WF, Labs SM, Casey DE (1987) Neuroleptic-induced Parkinsonism in older schizophrenics. Biol Psychiatry 22:427-439

Huber G (1957) Pneumencephalographische und psychopathologische Bilder bei endogenen Psychosen. Springer, Berlin Göttingen Heidelberg

Insel TR, Siever LJ (1981) The dopamine system challenge in affective disorders: a review of behavioral and neuroendocrine responses. J Clin Psychopharmacol 4:207-213

Johnstone EC, Crow TJ, Frith CD, Husband J, Kreel L (1976) Cerebral ventricular size and cognitive impairment in chronic schizophrenia. Lancet 2: 924-926

Johnstone EC, Crow TJ, Frith CD, Camey MWP, Price JS (1978) Mechanism of the antipsychotic effect in the treatment of acute schizophrenia. Lancet 1:848-851

Kaminski R, Powchick P, Warne PA, Goldstein M, McQueeney RT, Davidson M (1990) Measurement of plasma homovanillic acid concentration in schizophrenic patients. Prog Neuropsychopharmacol Biol Psychiatry 14:271-287

Kane JM, Honigfeld G, Singer J, Meltzer HY (1988) Clozapine for the treatment-resistant schizophrenic: a double-blind comparison versus chlorpromazine/benztropine. Arch Gen Psychiatry 48:789-796

Kay SR, Opler LA (1987) The positive-negative dimension in schizophrenia: its validity and significance. Psychiatr Dev 5:79-103

Kay SR, Opler LA, Fiszbein A (1987) Positive and negative syndrome scale (PANSS). Rating manual. Social and Behavioral Documents, San Rafael

Kendler KS, Heninger GR, Roth RH (1982a) Influence of dopamine agonists on plasma and brain levels of homovanillic acid. Life Sci 30:2063-2069

Kendler KS, Hsieh JYK, Davis KL (1982b) Studies of plasma homovanillic acid as an index of brain dopamine function. Psychopharmacol Bull 18:152-155

Kleinmann JE, Bridge P, Karoum F, Speciale S, Staub R, Zaleman S, Gillin JC, Wyatt RJ (1979) Catecholamines and metabolites in the brain of psychotics and normals: post mortem studies. In: Usdin E, Kopin IJ, Barchas J (eds) Catecholamines: brain and clinical frontiers. Pergamon, New York, pp 1845-1847

Kolivakis T, Azim H, Kingstone E (1974) A doubleblind comparison of pimozide and chlorpromazine in the maintenance care of chronic outpatients. Curr Ther Res 16:998-1004

König P, Benzer MK, Frische H (1991) SPECT technique for visualization of cerebral dopamine D_2 receptors. Am J Psychiatry 148:1607-1608

Kopin IJ (1992) Origin and significance of dopa and catecholamine metabolites in body fluids. Pharmacopsychiatry 25:333-336

Kornhuber J, Riederer P, Reynolds GP, Beckmann H, Jellinger K, Gabriel E (1989) ^{3}H-spiperone binding sites in post-mortem brains from schizophrenic patients: relationship to neuroleptic drug treatment, abnormal movements, and positive symptoms. J Neural Transm 75:1-10

Laux G, Klieser E, Schröder HG, Dittman V, Unterweger B, Schubert H, König P, Schöny HW, Bunse J, Beckmann H (1990) A double-blind multicenter study comparing remoxipride, two and three times daily, with haloperidol. Acta Psychiatr Scand 82 Suppl 358:125-129

Lewine RJ, Meltzer HY (1984) Negative symptoms and platelet monoamine oxidase activity in male schizophrenic patients. Psychiatry Res 12:99-109

Lewine RJ, Fogg L, Meltzer HY (1983) Assessment of negative and positive symptoms in schizophrenia. Schizophr Bull 9:368-376

Liddle PF (1987) The symptoms of chronic schizophrenia: a reexamination of the positive-negative dichotomy. Br J Psychiatry 151:145-151

Lieberman JA, Kane JM, Gadalletta D, Ramos-Lorenz J, Bergmann K, Wegner J, Novacenko H (1985) Methylphenidate challenge tests and course of schizophrenia. Psychopharmacol Bull 3: 111-121

Lindström LH (1985) Low HVA and normal 5-HIAA CSF levels in drug-free schizophrenic patients compared to healthy volunteers: correlations to symptomatology and family history. Psychiatry Res 14:265-273

Linnoila M, Ninan PT, Scheinin M, Waters RN, Chang WH, Barko J, van Kammen DP (1983) Reliability of norepinephrine and major monoamine metabolite measurements in CSF of schizophrenic patients. Arch Gen Psychiatry 40:1290-1294

Losonczy MF, Song IS, Mohs RC, Mathe AA, Davidson M, Davis BM, Davis KL (1986) Correlates of lateral ventricular size in chronic schizophrenia. II. Biological measures. Am J Psychiatry 143:1113-1118

Maas JW, Contreras SA, Bowden CL, Weintraub SE (1985) Effects of debrisoquin on CSF and plasma HVA concentrations in man. Life Sci 36:2163-2170

Maas JW, Contreras SA, Seleshi E, Bowden CL (1988) Dopamine metabolism and disposition in schizophrenic patients. Arch Gen Psychiatry 45:553-560

MacKay AVP (1981) Positive and negative schizophrenic symptoms and the role of dopamine. Br J Psychiatry 137:379–383
Maier W, Schlegel S, Klinger T, Hillert A, Wetzel H (1990) Die Negativsymptomatik im Verhältnis zur Positivsymptomatik und zur depressiven Symptomatik der Schizophrenie: Eine psychometrische Untersuchung. In: Möller H, Pelzer E (eds) Neuere Ansätze zur Diagnostik und Therapie schizophrener Minussymptomatik. Springer, Berlin Heidelberg New York, pp 69–78
Malas KL, van Kammen DP, Defraites EA, Brown GM, Gold PW (1983) Platelet monoamine oxidase and growth hormone response to apomorphine in schizophrenia. Biol Psychiatry 18:255–259
Malm U, Perris C, Rapp W, Wedren G (1974) A multicenter controlled trial of fluspirilene and fluphenazine enanthate in chronic schizophrenic syndromes. Acta Psychiatr Scand Suppl 249:94–116
Marder SR, Meibach RC (1994) Risperidone in the treatment of schizophrenia. Am J Psychiatrie 13:25–40
Martinot JL, Peron-Magnan P, Huret JD, Mazoyer B, Baron JC, Boulenger JP, Loc'h C, Maziere B, Caillard V, Loo H, Syrota A (1990) Striatal D_2-dopaminergic receptors assessed by positron emission tomography and ^{76}Br-bromospiperone in untreated schizophrenics. Am J Psychiatry 147:44–50
Martinot JL, Paillere-Martinot Ml, Loc'h C, Hardi P, Poirier MF, Mazoyer B, Beaufils B, Maziere B, Allilaire JF, Syrota A (1991) The estimated density of D_2 striatal receptors in schizophrenia. Br J Psychiatry 158:346–350
Mathieu P, Lemoine P, Szestak M, Greffe J, Gros N, Echassoux C (1985) Homovanillic acid urinary excretion and day/night rhythm of chronic schizophrenic patients. Preliminary observations. Encephale 11:199–202
Mayer-Gross W (1920) Über die Stellungnahme zur abgelaufenen akuten Psychose. Z Gesamte Neurol Psychiatr 60:160–212
Meltzer HJ, Kolakowska T, Fang VS, Fogg L, Robertson A, Lewine R, Strahilevitz M, Busch D (1984) Growth hormon and prolactin response to apomorphine in schizophrenia and the major affective disorders. Arch Gen Psychiatry 41:512–519
Meltzer HY (1985) Dopamine and negative symptoms in schizophrenia: critique of the type I-II hypothesis. In: Alpert M (ed) Controversies in schizophrenia. Guilford, New York, pp 110–136
Meltzer HY (1991) The effect of clozapine and other atypical antipsychotic drugs on negative symptoms. In: Mameros A, Andreasen, Tsuang MT (eds) Negative versus positive schizophrenia. Springer, Berlin Heidelberg New York, pp 365–376
Meltzer HY, Zureick J (1989) Negative symptoms in schizophrenia: a target for new drug development. In: Dahl SG, Gram LF (eds) Clinical pharmacology in psychiatry. Springer, Berlin Heidelberg New York, pp 68–77
Meltzer HY, Sommers AA, Luchins DJ (1986) The effect of neuroleptics and other psychotropic drugs on negative symptoms in schizophrenia. J Clin Psychopharmacol 6:329–338
Meltzer HY, Bastani B, Kwon KY, Ramirez LF, Burnett S, Sharpe J (1989) A prospective study of clozapine in treatment-resistant patients. I. Preliminary report. Psychopharmacology (Berl) 99 Suppl: 68–72
Miller R, Wickens JR, Beninger RJ (1990) Dopamine D-1 and D-2 receptors in relationship to reward and performance: a case for the D-1 receptor for the primary site of the therapeutic action of neuroleptic drugs. Prog Neurobiol 34:143–183
Möller HJ (1987) Konsequenzen aus der klinischen Psychopharmakologie für die nosologische und syndromatologische Klassifikation funktioneller psychischer Störungen. In: Simhandl C, Berner P, Luccioni H, Alf C (eds) Klassifikationsprobleme in der Psychiatrie. Medpharmazeutische Verlagsgesellschaft, Pukersdorf, pp 163–188
Möller HJ (1991) Typical neuroleptics in the treatment of positive and negative symptoms. In: Marneros A, Andreasen NC, Tsuang MT (eds) Negative versus positive schizophrenia. Springer, Berlin Heidelberg New York, pp 341–364
Möller HJ (1993) Neuroleptic treatment of negative symptoms in schizophrenic patients. Efficacy problems and methodological difficulties. Eur Neuropsychopharmacol 3:1–11
Möller HJ (1995) The psychopathology of schizophrenia: An integrated view of positive symptoms and negative symptoms. Int Clin Psychopharmacol (in press)
Möller HJ, von Zerssen D (1981) Depressive Symptomatik im stationären Behandlungsverlauf von 280 schizophrenen Patienten. Pharmakopsychiatria 14:172–179
Möller HJ, von Zerssen D (1982) Depressive states occurring during the neuroleptic treatment of schizophrenia. Schizophr Bull 8:109–117
Möller HJ, von Zerssen D (1986) Der Verlauf schizophrener Psychosen unter den gegenwärtigen Behandlungsbedingungen. Springer, Berlin Heidelberg New York

Möller HJ, van Praag HM, Aufdembrinke B et al. (1994) Negative symptoms in schizophrenia: considerations for clinical trials. Working group on negative symptoms in schizophrenia. Psychopharmacology (Berl) 15:221–228
Möller HJ, Müller H, Borison RL, Schooler NR, Chouinard G (1995) A path-analytical approach to differentiate between direct and indirect drug effect on negative symptoms in schizophrenic patients. A re-evaluation of the North American risperidone study. Eur Arch Psychiatry Clin Neurosci 245:45–49
Müller-Spahn F (1990) Die Bedeutung von Neuroleptika der neueren Generation in der Therapie schizophrener Patienten mit Minus-Symptomatik. In: Möller HJ, Pelzer E (eds) Neuere Ansätze zur Diagnostik und Therapie schizophrener Minussymptomatik. Springer, Berlin Heidelberg New York, pp 207–215
Müller-Spahn F (1991) Diagnostik und Therapie schizophrener Minus-Symptomatik. Schnetztor, Konstanz
Müller-Spahn F, Ackenheil M, Albus M, Kurtz G (1987) Neuroendokrinologische Untersuchungen bei schizophrenen Patienten nach Stimulation mit unterschiedlichen Dosierungen von Apomorphin. In: Beckmann H, Laux G (eds) Biologische Psychiatrie. Springer, Berlin Heidelberg New York, pp 117–121
Newcomer JW, Riney SJ, Vinogradov S, Csernansky JG (1992) Plasma prolactin and homovanillic acid as markers for psychopathology and abnormal movements during maintenance haloperidol treatment in male patients with schizophrenia. Psychiatry Res 41:191–202
Nybäck H, Bergen BM, Hindmarsh T, Sedvall G, Wiesel F (1983) Cerebroventricular size and cerebrospinal fluid monoamine metabolites in schizophrenic patients and healthy volunteers. Psychiatry Res 9:301–308
Pandurangi AK, Bilder RM, Rieder RO, Mukherjee S, Hamer RM (1988) Schizophrenic symptoms and deterioration. Relation to computed tomographic findings. J Nerv Ment Dis 176: 200–206
Papeschi R, McClure DJ (1971) Homovanillic and 5-hydroxyindoleacetic acid in cerebrospinal fluid in depressed patients. Arch Gen Psychiatry 25:354–358
Persson T, Roos BE (1969) Acid metabolites from monoamines in cerebrospinal fluid of schizophrenics. Br J Psychiatry 115:95–98
Peselow ED, Stanley M (1982) Clinical trials of benzamides in psychiatry. Adv Biochem Psychopharmacol 35:163–194
Pickar D, Labarca R, Doran A, Wolkowitz OM, Roy A, Breier A, Linnoila M, Paul SM (1986) Longitudinal measurement of plasma homovanillic acid levels in schizophrenic patients. Arch Gen Psychiatry 43:669–676
Pickar D, Wolkowitz OM, Doran AR, Labarca R, Roy A, Breier A, Narang PK (1987) Clinical and biochemical effects of verapamil administration to schizophrenic patients. Arch Gen Psychiatry 44:113–118
Pilc A, Ventulani J (1982) Depression by chronic electroconvulsive treatment of clonidine hypothermia and clonidine binding to rat cortical membrane. Eur J Pharmacol 80:109–113
Piletz JE, Schubert DSP, Halaris A (1986) Evaluation of studies on platelet alpha-2-adrenoreceptors in depressive illness. Life Sci 39:1589–1616
Piletz JE, Halaris A, Saran A, Maler M (1991) Desipramine lowers ^{3}H-p-aminoclonidine binding in platelets of depressed patients. Arch Gen Psychiatry 48:813–820
Pinder RM, Brogden RN, Sawyer PR et al. (1976) Pimozide: a review of its pharmacological properties and therapeutic uses in psychiatry. Drugs 12:1–40
Post RM, Fink E, Carpenter WT Jr, Goodwin FK (1975) Cerebrospinal fluid amine metabolites in acute schizophrenia. Arch Gen Psychiatry 32:1063–1069
Potkin SG, Weinberger DR, Linnoila M, Wyatt RJ (1983) Low CSF 5-hydroxyindoleacetic acid in schizophrenic patients with enlarged cerebral ventricles. Am J Psychiatry 140:21–25
Prosser ES, Csemansky JG, Kaplan H, Thiemann S, Becker TJ, Hollister LE (1987) Depression, Parkinsonian symptoms, and negative symptoms in schizophrenics treated with neuroleptics. J Nerv Ment Dis 175:100–105
Rao ML, Möller HJ (1994) Biochemical findings of negative symptoms in schizophrenia and their putative relevance to pharmacologic treatment. Pharmacopsychiatry 30:160–172
Rao VAR, Bailey J, Bishop M, Coppen A (1981) A clinical and pharmacodynamic evaluation of sulpiride. Psychopharmacology 73: 77–80
Reubenstein M, Schindler AF, Gershanik O, Stefano FJE (1989) Positive interaction between alpha-1 adrenergic and dopamine-2 receptors in locomotor activity of normo- and supersensitive mice. Life Sci 44:337–346
Rimon R, Roos BE, Rakkolainen V, Alanen Y (1971) The content of 5-HIAA and HVA in the CSF of patients with acute schizophrenia. J Psychosom Res 15:375–378

Rosen J, Silk KR, Rice HE, Smith CB (1985) Platelet alpha-2-adrenergic dysfunction in negative symptom schizophrenia: a preliminary study. Biol Psychiatry 20:539–545

Rösler M, Hengesch G (1990) 'Negative' symptoms im AMDP-system. In: Baum U, Fähndrich E, Stieglitz RD, Woggon B (eds) Veränderungsmessung in Psychiatrie und Klinischer Psychologie. Profil, Munich, pp 329–339

Seeman P (1987) Dopamine receptors and the dopamine hypothesis of schizophrenia. Synapse 1:133–152

Smith CB, Garcia-Sevilla JA, Hollingsworth PJ (1981) Alpha-adrenoreceptors in rat brain are decreased after long-term tricyclic antidepressant drug treatment. Brain Res 210:413–418

Snyder SH (1972) Catecholamines in the brain as mediators of amphetamine psychosis. Arch Gen Psychiatry 27:169–179

Sommers AA (1985) 'Negative symptoms': conceptual and methodological problems. Schizophr Bull 11:364–379

Stein L, Wise CD (1971) Possible etiology of schizophrenia: progressive damage to the noradrenergic reward system by 6-hydroxydopamine. Science 171:1032–1036

Steinberg JL, Garver DL, Moeller FG, Raese JD, Orsulak PF (1993) Serum homovanillic acid levels in schizophrenic patients and normal control subjects. Psychiatry Res 48:93–106

Strauss JS, Carpenter WT Jr, Bartko JJ (1974) The diagnosis and understanding of schizophrenia. III. Speculations on the processes that underline schizophrenic symptoms and signs. Schizophr Bull 1:61–69

Swerdlow NR, Koob GF (1989) Norepinephrine stimulates behavioral activation in rats following depletion of nucleus accumbens dopamine. Pharmacol Biochem Behav 33:595–599

van der Heyden P, Ebinger G, Kanarek L (1986) Vanquelin, epinephrine and norepinephrine stimulation of adenylate cyclase in bovine retina homogenate: evidence for interaction with the D_1-receptor. Life Sci 38:1221–1228

van Kammen DP, Boronow JJ (1988) Dextro-amphetamine diminishes negative symptoms in schizophrenia. Int Clin Psychopharmacol 3:111–121

van Kammen DP, Antelman S (1984) Impaired noradreneric transmission in schizophrenia? Life Sci 34:1403–1413

van Kammen DP, Mann LS, Sternberg DE, Scheinin M, Ninan PT, Marder SR, van Kammen WB, Rieder RO, Linnoila M (1983) Dopamine β-hydroxylase activity and homovanillic acid in spinal fluid of patients with brain atrophy. Science 220:974–977

van Kammen DP, Hommer DW, Malas KL (1987) Effect of pimozide on positive and negative symptoms in schizophrenic patients: are negative symptoms state dependent? Neuropsychobiology 18:113–117

van Kammen DP, Mouton A, Kelley M, Breeding W, Peters J (1991) Exploration of dopamine and noradrenaline activity and negative symptoms in schizophrenia: concepts and controversies. In: Marneros A, Andreasen NC, Tsuang MT (eds) Negative versus positive schizophrenia. Springer, Berlin Heidelberg New York, pp 317–340

van Praag HM, Korf J (1973) Cerebral monoamines and depression: an investigation with the probenecid technique. Arch Gen Psychiatry 28:827–831

Waddington JL, Youssef HA, Molloy AG, O'Boyle KM, Pugh MT (1985) Association of intellectual impairment, negative symptoms, and aging with tardive dyskinesia: clinical and animal studies. J Clin Psychiatry 46:29–33

Wing JK (1978) Clinical concepts of schizophrenia. In: Wing JK (ed) Schizophrenia: toward a new synthesis. Academic, London, pp 1–30

Woggon B (1990) Wirkprofile klassischer Neuroleptika und die Beeinflussung von Minussymptomatik. In: Möller HJ, Pelzer E (eds) Neuere Ansätze zur Diagnostik und Therapie schizophrener Minussymptomatik. Springer, Berlin Heidelberg New York, pp 199–205

Wong DF, Wagner HN Jr, Tune LE, Dannals RF, Pearlson GD, Links JM, Tamminga CA, Broussole EP, Raver HT, Wilson AA, Toung JKT, Malat J, Williams JA, O'Tuama LA, Snyder SH, Kuhar MJ, Gjedde A (1986) Positron emission tomography reveals elevated D_2 dopamine receptors in drug-naive schizophrenics. Science 234:1558–1563

Zemlan FP, Hischowitz J, Garver DL (1986) Relation of clinical symptoms to apomorphin stimulated growth hormone release in mood incongruent psychotic patients. Arch Gen Psychiatry 43:1162–1167

Zinner HJ, Kraemer S, Möller HJ (1990) Empirische Untersuchungen zur Konkordanz verschiedener Minus-Symptomatik-Skalen sowie zur Korrelation mit testpsychologischen Befunden. In: Möller HJ, Pelzer E (eds) Neuere Ansätze zur Diagnostik und Therapie schizophrener Minussymptomatik. Springer, Berlin Heidelberg New York, pp 59–68

Interaction of Long-Term Antidepressant Treatment with Psychosocial Factors

F. Bauwens, D. Pardoen, and J. Mendlewicz

Introduction

Longitudinal studies on the long-term course of bipolar and unipolar affective disorders have demonstrated a rather high rate of recurrences, even in patients maintained on lithium or antidepressant prophylaxis (Prien 1987). Numerous investigations have attempted to identify predictors and triggering factors of the recurrences. Although a role for biological and genetic factors has been strongly suggested (Mendlewicz 1972; Mendlewicz et al. 1984), the study of environmental and psychosocial variables has also been shown to be of interest in the prediction of the long-term course of bipolar and unipolar affective illness. In particular, research has focused on the impact of life events on onset of affective episodes and on several psycho-social characteristics of depressive patients, such as self-esteem, social adjustment and social support. Thus, a large body of studies has shown a consistent association between stressful life events and onset of affective episodes in both community and patient samples (Favarelli 1987). However, in spite of its consistency this association was rather limited (explaining about 10 % of the variance), in line with the common observation that a large proportion of persons who experience stressfull life events do not become clinically depressed. Research has thus attempted to define other psychosocial risk factors that could mediate the relationship between life events and depression. The availability of a supportive social network was identified as a potential protective factor against depression (O'Connel et al. 1991; Brugha et al. 1990) while a low or fragile self-esteem was emphasized as increasing liability to depression (Ingham et al. 1987). Furthermore, various social maladjustments which classically accompany depressive states appeared to persist after remission (Weissman et al. 1981) and were hypothesized as playing a role in the predisposition towards subsequent episodes (Coyne 1976). So far, few studies have selected clinically homogenous samples. It has been shown that the impact of life events is greater at the beginning of the affective illness than on later recurrences (Ezquiaga et al. 1987; Ghaziuddin et al. 1990) but recent studies by Frank et al. (1994) and Brown et al. (1994) observed that life events may play a role in triggering recurrences characterized by nonendogenous features.

Post (1992) has developed the *kindling model*, which postulates that affective illness has an increasingly autonomous course linked to a sensitization to both stressors and episodes. Another hypothesis concerning the smaller role of life events on recurrences has been stressed by Sclare and Creed (1990), who argue that the progression of the affective disorders is frequently accompanied by an impoverishment of usual work and recreational activities which lead to a reduced exposure to life events.

It is to note that most of the above studies were either retrospectively conducted or initiated during the depressive state, leaving some doubt on the episode independence of the psychosocial predictors or triggering factors. The present investigation assessed psychosocial and clinical variables in a longitudinal one-year design with patients in remission for at least 6 months at inclusion into the study.

Subjects and Methods

The study was conducted between 1986 and 1989 in the out-patient clinic of the psychiatric department of our university hospital. Patient sample consised in 27 bipolar patients and 25 unipolar patients, diagnosed on the basis of the Schedule for affective Disorders and Schizophrenia (SADS, Endicott and Spitzer 1978), according to the Research Diagnostic Criteria (RDC, Spitzer et al. 1978). Patients had to be free of any other RDC diagnoses and of any concurrent severe physical illness. At time of entry into the study, they had to have at least a 6-month period of remission, defined according to RDC criteria as the absence of manic (definite or probable), hypomanic (definite), major depressive (definite or probable) and minor depressive (definite) episodes. Rapid cyders were excluded. A healthy control group included 26 subjects selected to have no personal or family history of psychiatric disorders (RDC) nor any current physical illness. The three groups were matched for age (mean = 46.64; range = 19–68), sex (38% male; 62% female), socioeconomic status (assessed with the Index of Social Position, Hollingshead and Redlich (1958): mean = 2.7, range = 1–5) and marital status (74% married or cohabiting, 26% single, widowed or divorced).

Prophylactic medication, started at least 1 year before entry into the study, consisted of lithium (900 mg/day, n = 25) or lithium and carbamazepine (n = 2) for bipolars and MAOI (phenelzine 30 mg/day, n = 1) or heterocydic antidepressant (amitriptyline 200 mg/day, n = 15; clomipramine 75 mg/day, n = 3; doxepine 75 mg/day, n = 2; desipramine 50 mg/day, n = 1; mianserine 30 mg/day, n = 1; nortriptyline 50 mg/day, n = 1) for unipolars. Blood samples were drawn every 2 months for the duration of the study in order to control medication compliance. Lithium regimen were adapted in order to achieve plasma level ranging from 0,6 to 1.2 mEq/liter. Full details of the sample population are provided in our earlier publication (Bauwens et al. 1991).

Instruments and Procedures

Throughout the 1-year study, subjects were seen every 2 months by a psychiatrist who assessed current mood state with the Hamilton Rating Scale for Depression (HDRS-17, Hamilton 1960) and symptom status since the last visit using the RDC (Spitzer et al. 1978). When an affective episode was diagnosed, its beginning was precisely dated. Subjects were also bimonthly seen by a clinical psychologist who assessed, blind to the patient's condition, the life events in the 2 previous months with the Interview for Recent Life Events (IRLE, Paykel and Mangen 1983), the social adjustment in various areas with the Social Adjustment Scale (SAS, Weissman and Paykel 1974), the self-esteem with the Rosenberg Self-Esteem Scale (RSE, Rosenberg 1965) and the social support with the Social Support Network Inventory (SSNI, Flaherty et al. 1983).

Statistical Analyses

Cross-sectional psychosocial variables were analysed using one-factor and two-factor analyses of variance. Their relationship with cross-sectional clinical variables was evaluated using Pearson correlations. The cumulative probability of recurrence by time since the beginning of the study was estimated by the Kaplan-Meier method. Life table analyses were used to evaluate the association between cross-sectional variables and recurrences. A generalised Savage-Mantel-Cox procedure was used in each group to compare life table curves. We performed t tests paired to look for variations of social adjustment scores in the 2 months preceding the affective episodes. Finally, to evaluate the temporal patterning of marked or severe life events in relation to episode onset, we used an adaptation of the Kaplan-Meier survival analysis, setting the date of episode onset as month 0 and working backward to the closest marked or severe life event.

Results

Psychosocial Variables at Entry into the Study

Comparison of social adjustment basic scores between the three groups of subjects showed an overall social maladjustment and, specifically, an impairement in social and leisure activities in the two groups of patients as compared to controls ($F = 15.09$; $df = 2$; $p < 0.001$). We also identified a marital maladjustment ($F = 3.92$; $df = 2$, $p < 0.05$) in unipolar patients. Focusing the analyses on self-esteem scores, we found that unipolars had a significantly lower self-esteem than both bipolars and controls ($F = 5.67$, $df = 2$, $p < 0.01$). No diffierences appeared between the scores of social support network for bipolars, unipolars and controls. In unipolar patients, no significant correlation was found between psychosocial and clinical variables. In contrast, bipolars' social maladjustments were significantly correlated to their mean number of lifetime affective episodes ($r = 0.40$, $p < 0.05$) and to their current residual symptomatology measured with HRSD-17 ($r = 0.47$, $p < 0.05$).

Course of Illness

During the study, two bipolars and six unipolars suffered a major depressive episode; 11 bipolars, 16 unipolars and six controls had a minor depressive episode; two bipolars presented a manic episode an four others had an hypomanic episode. Due to sample size and the small number of major recurrences, major and minor recurrences had to be grouped in order to perform statistical tests. The subjects who remained euthymic during the study were 11 bipolars, five unipolars and 20 controls. Those who met, at minimum, the criteria for an episode of minor severity (minor or major depressive, hypomanic or manic definite episode) were 16 bipolars, 19 unipolars and six controls.

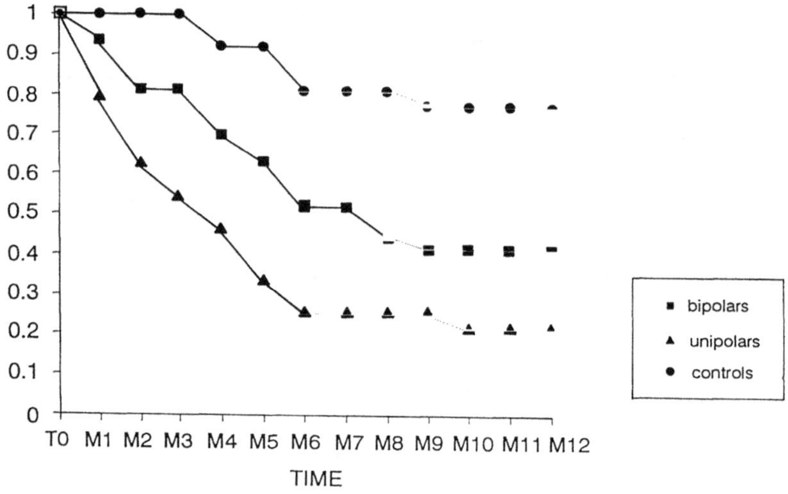

Fig. 1. Cumulative proportions of subjects remaining without major or minor affective recurrences

According to this definition of affective episode, Mantel-Cox analysis comparing survival curves between the three groups of subjects, showed a consistent tendancy for bipolars to be more at risk than controls ($p < 0.05$) and for unipolars to be more at risk than bipolars ($p < 0.05$) and controls ($p < 0.01$) (Fig. 1).

Predictors of Recurrences

A series of Mantel-Cox analyses was performed to evaluate the association between cross-sectional variables, dichotomized according to the median, and time to recurrences. Work adjustment appeared to be the strongest predictor of recurrences in both bipolar ($p > 0.01$) and unipolar patients ($p < 0.05$) (Fig. 2). Moreover, adjustment in social and leisure activities ($p < 0.01$) and selfesteem ($p < 0.05$) predicted affective recurrences in bipolar patients while several aspects of marital adjustment ($p < 0.05$) predicted unipolars' depressive recurrences. Clinical characteristics assessed at entry into the study appeared to be less related to the occurrence of affective recurrences during the 1-year period. The only predictors identified were HRSD-17 baseline scores in bipolars ($p < 0.05$) and history of endogenous depression for unipolars ($p < 0.05$).

Changes in Psychosocial Variables Before Recurrences

A series of paired t tests were performed comparing, in each group, the social adjustment and self-esteem scores in the 2 months preceding the affective episodes with the scores rated at the beginning of the study. No significant changes were found in the scores of patients and controls.

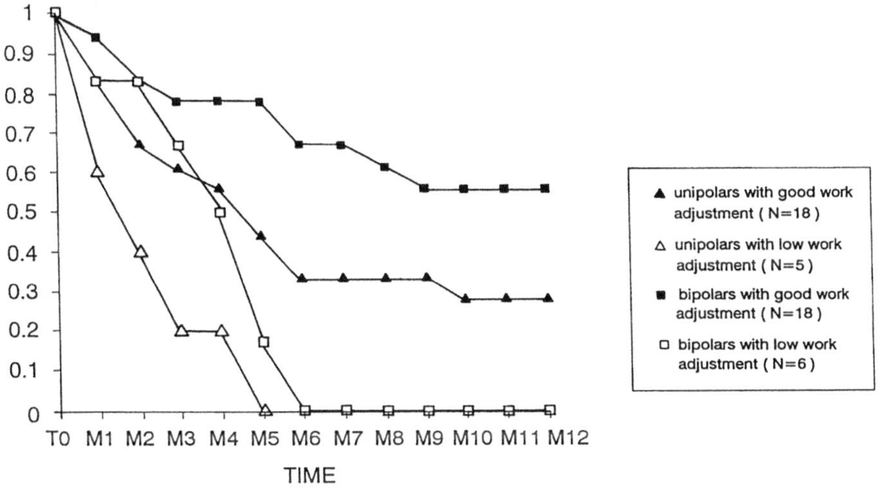

Fig. 2. Cumulative proportions of bipolars and unipolars remaining without major or minor affective episodes given their global level of work adjustment

Temporal Patterning of Marked or Severe Events Before Recurrences

As shown in Fig. 3 and 4, in both bipolar and unipolar patients, the survival time from the occurrence of a marked or severe life event to onset of a recurrence was not significantly different than for patients having not suffered an affective recurrence during a similar matched period of observation. Conversely, in the control group, survival analysis revealed a significant difference between subjects having or not having experienced a minor depressive episode (Fig. 5).

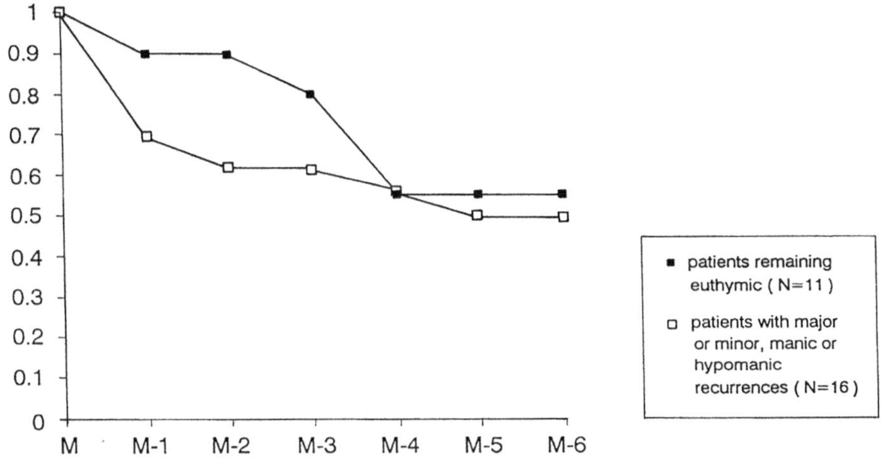

Fig. 3. Cumulative probability of no marked or severly threatening life event in bipolar patients

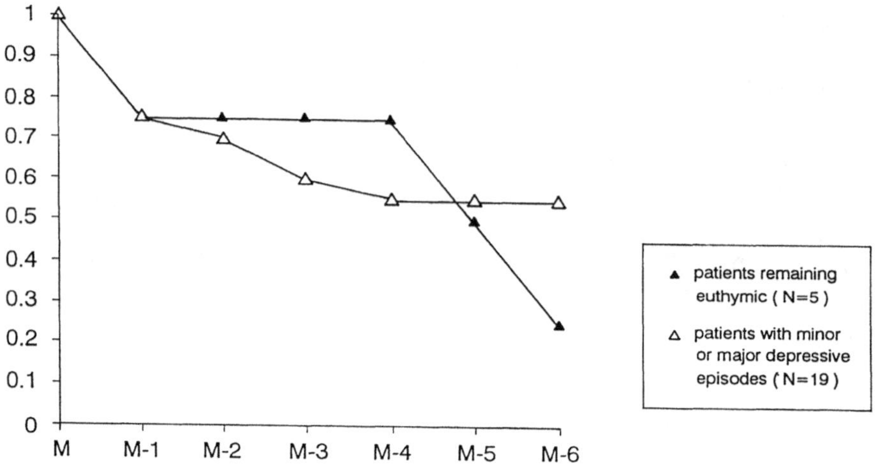

Fig. 4. Cumulative probability of no marked or severely threatening life event in unipolar patients

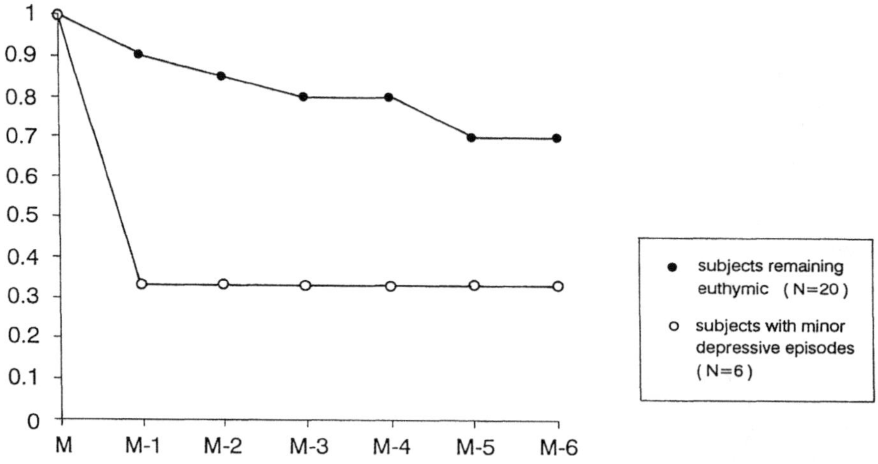

Fig. 5. Cumulative probability of no marked or severely threatening life event in control subjects

Discussion

Comparisons of psychosocial variables at entry into the study showed, in both groups of recovered patients, the persistence of a mild social maladjustment, particularly affecting the area of social and leisure activities. Unipolars appeared more impaired than bipolars: they had a specific dysfunctioning in marital relationships and a lower self-esteem than bipolars and healthy controls. These results are in line with several studies on social adjustment (Weissman et al. 1981) and self-esteem (Ingham et al. 1987) after recovery from a major depressive episode. The less impaired profile found for our bipolar patients could be related to their tendency to conform socially and behave conventionally, as described by earlier studies (Matussek and Feil 1983), or to the effect of lithium prophylaxis. Surprisingly, the social support network of our bipolar and unipolar recovered patients did not differ from that of healthy controls. This finding is at variance with studies having shown that, after remission from a major depressive episode, patients continued to experience smaller and less supportive social networks than did control subjects without psychiatric history (Gotlib and Lee 1989). This discrepancy could be attributed to the absence, in these studies, of a remission period required before investigation, which did not allow avoidance of cognitive bias linked to the previous depressive episode.

During the 1-year period of investigation, we observed a 14% rate of major affective episodes in bipolar patients and a 25% rate of major depressive episodes in unipolar patients. This result is in line with longitudinal studies in bipolars on lithium or carbamazepine prophylaxis (Goodwin and Jamison 1990) and in unipolars maintained on antidepressant treatment (Shea et al. 1992; Kupfer et al. 1992). Our rather high rate of minor recurrences may be compared to prospective studies on subsyndromal symptoms in bipolars (Goodnick et al. 1987) and unipolars (Maj et al. 1992) maintained on prophylactic treatment. Several psychosocial baseline variables appeared to be relevant in the prediction of recurrences. In particular, work adjustment predicted recurrences in both groups of patients; difficulties in marital relationships were associated with recurrences in unipolars; low self-esteem and impaired social and leisure activities forecasted the occurrence of new affective episodes in bipolar patients. Conversely, most characteristics of illness history did not predict recurrences during the 1-year period of investigation. Only history of endogenous episodes was associated with time to depressive recurrences in unipolars. Furthermore, residual symptomatology measured at entry into the study predicted further episodes in bipolar patients. These results confirm studies showing psychosocial variables as risk factors of affective episodes (Hirschfeld and Cross 1982). However, these variables were not found to deteriorate in the 2-month period preceding the recurrences and recent life events did not appear to trigger recurrences in either bipolar or unipolar patients. Thus, the course of recurrent affective disorders seems to be more related to long-standing psychosocial difficulties rather than to recent problems. This observation is in keeping with several studies which have shown the greater impact of life events at the onset of both bipolar and unipolar illness than on later recurrences (Perris 1984; Ezquiaga et al. 1987). Further research is indicated to evaluate how clinical management strategies may address these long-term psychosocial difficulties and contribute to the prophylaxis of affective disorders.

Acknowledgements: The research was supported by the Fonds National de la Recherche Scientifique, the Association pour l'Etude de la Santé Mentale, the Biomedical and Health Research Project from the European Commission and the Ministère de la Communauté Française. We are very grateful to A. Tracy, M.Sc. for assessments of social adjustment and to M. Vanderelst, M.D. and A. Vilane, M.D. for psychiatric screening of subjects. Our thanks also go to E. Braeckman and C. Plees for technical assistance.

References

Bauwens F et al. (1991) Social adjustment of remitted bipolar and unipolar out-patients. A comparison with age- and sex-matched controls. Br J Psychiatry 159:239–244
Brown GW, Harris TO, Hepworth C (1994) Life events and endogenous depression: a puzzle reexamined. Arch Gen Psychiatry 51:525–534
Brugha TS, Bebbington PE, McCarthy B, Sturt T, Wykes T, Potter J (1990) Gender, social support and recovery from depressive disorders: a prospective clinical study. Psychol Med 20:147–156
Coyne JC (1976) Toward an interactional description of depression. Psychiatry 39:28–40
Endicott J, Spitzer RL (1978) A diagnostic interview: the schedule for affective disorders and schizophrenia. Arch Gen Psychiatry 35:837–844
Ezquiaga E, Gutierrez JLA, Lopez AG (1987) Psychosocial factors and episode number in depression. J Affective Disord 12:135–138
Ingham JG, Kreitman NB, Miller PMM, Sadisharan SP (1978) Self-appraisal, anxiety and depression in women: a prospective enquiry. Br J Psychiatry 142:247–256
Favarelli C, Pallanti S, Frassine R et al. (1987) Life events and depression. In: Racagni G, Smeraldi E (eds) Anxious depression: assess and treatment. Raven, New York
Flaherty JA, Gaviria FM, Black EM et al. (1983) The role of social support in the functioning of patients unipolar depression. Am J Psychiatry 140 (4):473–476
Frank E, Anderson B, Reynolds CF III, Ritenour A, Kupfer D (1994) Life events and the Research Diagnostic Criteria Endogenous Subtype. Arch Gen Psychiatry 51:519–524
Ghaziuddin M, Ghaziuddin N, Stein GS (1990) Life events and the recurrence of depression. Can J Psychiatry 35:239–242
Goodnick PJ, Fieve RR, Schlegel A, Kaufman K (1987) Inter-episode major and subclinical symptoms in affective disorder. Acta Psychiatr Scand 75:597–600
Goodwin F, Jamison K (1990) Manic-depressive illness. Oxford University Press, New York
Gotlib I, Lee C (1989) The social functioning of depressed patients: a longitudinal assessment. J Soc clin Psychol 8:223–237
Hamilton M (1960) A rating scale for depression. J Neurol Neurosurg Psychiatry 23:17–19, 56–62
Hirschfeld RM, Cross CK (1982) Epidemiology of affective disorders, psychosocial risk factors Arch Gen Psychiatry 39:35–46
Hollingshead AB, Redlich FC (1958) Social class and mental illness. Wiley New York
Kupfer DJ, Frank E, Perel JM, Cornes C, Mallinger AG, Thase ME, McEachran AB, Grochocinski VJ (1992) Five-year outcome of maintenance therapies in recurrent depression. Arch Gen Psychiatry 49:769–773
Maj M, Veltro F, Pirozzi R, Lobrace S, Magliano L (1992) Pattern of recurrence of illness after recovery from an episode of major depression: a prospective study. Am J Psychiatry 149:795–800
Matussek P, Feil WB (1983) Personality attributes of depressive patients. Arch Gen Psychiatry 40:783–790
Mendlewicz J (1972) The nature of affective equivalents in relation to affective disorders. Excerpta Med Int Congr Ser 274:638–643
Mendlewicz J, Kerkhofs M, Hoffman G, Linkowski P (1984) Dexamethasone suppression test and Rem sleep in patients with major depressive disorder. Br J Psychiatry 145:383–388
O'Connel RA, Mayo JA, Flatow L, Cuthbertson B, O'Brien BE (1991) Outcome of bipolar disorder in long-term treatment with lithium. Br J Psychiatry 159:123–129
Pardoen D et al. (1993) Self-esteem in recovered bipolar and unipolar out-patients. Br J Psychiatry 163:755–762
Paykel ES, Mangen SP (1983) Interview for recent life events. J Psychosom Res 27:341–521
Perris H (1984) Life events and depression. II. Results in diagnostic subgroups and in relation to recurrence in depression. J Affective Disord 7:25–36
Post RM (1992) Transduction of psychosocial stress into the neurobiology of recurrent affective disorder. Am J Psychiatry 149 (8):999–1010
Prien RF (1987) Long-term treatment of affective disorders. In: Meltzer HY (ed) Psychopharmacology: the third generation of progress. Raven, New York, pp 1051–1058
Rosenberg M (1965) Society and the adolescent self-image. Princeton University Press, Princeton
Sclare P, Creed F (1990) Life events and the onset of mania. Br J Psychiatry 156:508–514
Shea MT, Elkin I, Imber SD et al. (1992) Course of depressive symptoms over follow-up: findings from the National Institute of Mental Health Treatment of Depression Collaborative Research Program. Arch Gen Psychiatry 49:782–787

Spitzer RL et al. (1978) Research diagnostic criteria for a selected group of functional disorders, 3rd edn. New York State Psychiatric Institute, Biometrics Research Division, New York
Weissman MM et al. (1981) Depressed outpatients. Arch Gen Psychiatry 38:51–55
Weissman MM, Klerman GL, Paykel ES (1974) Treatment effects on the social adjustment of depressed outpatients. Arch Gen Psychiatry 30:771–778